POUNDS
OFF

PREVENTION'S

FAMILY HEALTH LIBRARY™

POUNDS OFF

Fast and Easy Weight Control and Fitness

by the Editors of
Prevention® Magazine

 Rodale Press, Emmaus, Pa.

Printed in the United States of America on recycled paper containing a high percentage of de-inked fiber.

Library of Congress Cataloging in Publication Data

Pounds off.

    (Prevention's family health library)
     1. Reducing diets.   2. Reducing.   3. Health.
I. Prevention (Emmaus, Pa.) II. Series.
RM222.2.P68   1987   613.2′5   86-31384
ISBN 0-87857-706-8   paperback

2   4   6   8   10   9   7   5   3   1   paperback

NOTICE

    This book is intended as a reference volume only, not as a medical manual or guide to self-treatment. If you suspect that you have a medical problem, we urge you to seek competent medical help. Keep in mind that nutritional and health needs vary from person to person, depending on age, sex, health status and total diet. The information here is intended to help you make informed decisions about your health, not as a substitute for any treatment that may have been prescribed by your doctor.

Contents

Contents

CHAPTER 1

Success Secrets of 5 Leading Diets

What if you selected some of the world's best health diets, fed detailed information about them into a computer and programmed it to find the crucial factors common to them all? What kind of news would come jumping off the printout?

Perhaps very good news indeed. For you could end up with a distillation of prime dietary principles, the essence of all the regimens with the nuances boiled off. Instead of a new brand-name diet, you'd have something bigger and better—guidelines that could be applied to any situation in any household.

To prove that such a distillation is feasible, we offer the following dietary signposts derived from five top health diets.

We found that even among this highly diverse collection of regimens, there's a common core of nutritional good sense. Here are the diets we distilled.

The American Heart Association Diet

This conservative regimen is probably the medical establishment's model for dietary prudence. It's part of the AHA's arsenal for fighting heart disease, so its main features are moderate cutbacks in the substances that contribute to the malady—fat, cholesterol, animal proteins and sodium.

Says an AHA spokesman, "The diet contains a lot of fruits and vegetables. And there's also an emphasis on balance to ensure that you get the proper amount of nutrients."

The Pritikin Diet

This is the controversial spartan regime developed by the late Nathan Pritikin, outspoken proponent of better nutrition and author of *The Pritikin Promise* (Simon and Schuster). Like the AHA diet, this dietary plan is seen as an answer to the degenerative diseases that ravage the American people—and an indictment of the same dietary factors that the AHA maligns. Pritikin's diet, however, doesn't feature moderate reductions in these substances, but drastic ones. Some doctors have criticized such nutritional austerity, but several recently published studies demonstrate the diet's power to reduce the symptoms of diabetes, high blood pressure and heart disease. Said Pritikin, "The diet consists of whole grains, legumes if you want, fruits, vegetables, nonfat dairy products and limited amounts of animal protein—about 1½ pounds per week. We exclude egg yolks, butter, margarine, oils, nuts, seeds and caffeine."

The Golden Door Diet

When luminaries from stage, screen and bookrack visit the famous Golden Door Spa in Escondido, California, this is the dietary scheme they embrace. It's the creation of the spa's founder, Deborah Szekely, author of *Golden Door Cookbook, The Greening of American Cuisine* (Golden Door).

Her approach is to try to fuse maximum food enjoyment with high-quality nutrition, a kind of sensible hedonism. With the zeal of a gourmet, she lauds the use of fresh fruits, fresh vegetables, fresh eggs, fresh everything. No processed foods allowed. And with the concern of a nutrition-minded doctor, she decries the typical American diet and insists on meals with less salt, no sugar and no red meat.

"Seafood is eaten three or four times a week," Szekely says. "Chicken once a week. Then there are meals relying on tofu, legumes, cheese, eggs. At lunch and dinner you must have some form of complete protein, but not in the quantity once thought necessary."

The "Aerobic Nutrition" Diet

"When there is just enough oxygen to permit the body to function and get by, but not enough to enable the body to enjoy its maximum capacity for good health, you can expect trouble. There is a direct relationship of nutrition to the availability of oxygen in the blood. That's what the term *aerobic nutrition* is all about."

So says the originator of this diet of aerobic efficiency, Don Mannerberg, M.D., a Dallas physician and co-author of *Aerobic Nutrition* (Hawthorn/Dutton). He points out that triglycerides—those insidious dietary fats—can slowly choke off the body's oxygen supply. One remedy is aerobic exercise. Another is aerobic eating, a dietary ploy to cut the triglycerides. To Dr. Mannerberg that means shunning foods high in fat, staying away from alcohol and caffeine, and avoiding single-meal gorging—the habit of skipping breakfast and eating big evening meals.

This dietary blueprint differs from the others not so much in content, but in degree. Somewhere between the asceticism of the Pritikin diet and the less stringent requirements of the AHA diet lies Dr. Mannerberg's regimen.

The Vegetarian Diet

In the United States the meatless regime is embraced by only a health-conscious or ethically concerned minority, but worldwide it is practiced by millions.

Says Dean Ornish, M.D., author of *Stress, Diet and Your Heart* (Holt, Rinehart and Winston), "It is still the way that most of the world eats—except for the industrialized countries like ours, where coronary heart disease is epidemic."

There may be as many as 200 different versions of the diet, but most vegetarians stick to either the vegan, lacto or lacto-ovo variety. The vegan menu consists of grains, legumes, nuts, fruits and vegetables. The lacto version incorporates milk, cheese and butter in this mix. And the lacto-ovo adds eggs as well.

At any rate, the common denominator, of course, is the absence of flesh foods. And that usually means a diet low in fat and high in complex carbohydrates and fiber.

Now let's get to the operating principles that make these diets work.

1. Eat Lean for Life

The AHA, Pritikin, Szekely, Dr. Mannerberg, Dr. Ornish—they all say what you've already guessed: Any diet worth a darn must be low in cholesterol and fat. There's simply too much evidence against this dangerous duo to suggest otherwise.

Dr. Ornish: "By now most informed medical people know that excessive fat and cholesterol in the body have been highly correlated with heart disease, colon cancer, breast cancer and a host of other ills. And there's no doubt that most people get the excess from the foods they eat."

Dr. Mannerberg: "Medical evidence indicates that the fat level in the usual American diet—amounting to 42 percent of total calories—is way too high. And the same goes for cholesterol."

So how low is low enough? It seems that in the realm of low-cholesterol, low-fat diets, there's plenty of room to experiment. The AHA regime allows 30 to 35 percent of your calories to be fat and permits cholesterol consumption of as much as 300 milligrams a day. At the other extreme are the Pritikin restrictions: only 5 to 10 percent of calories in fat and no more than 100 milligrams of cholesterol daily. Between these benchmarks you'll encounter the fat and cholesterol levels of the Golden Door, Dr. Mannerberg, and perhaps even a few vegetarian regimens.

According to the AHA, its requirements imply only minimal changes in standard meals and menus. You limit egg yolks to three a week; go easy on shrimp and organ meats; consume more fish, chicken and turkey than beef, lamb and pork; substitute vegetable protein for meat whenever you can; and use two to four tablespoons of polyunsaturated oil or margarine daily.

Pushing fat and cholesterol intake down to Pritikin levels, however, requires more discipline. To toe the line you'll need to keep that weekly 1½ pounds of animal protein as lean as possible and eat a daily ration of two or more kinds of whole grain, four or more servings of fresh vegetables (at least two of which must be raw) and four servings of fresh fruit. Sweet potatoes, squash and legumes are optional, and honey and sugar are banned right along with egg yolks and fatty dairy products.

2. Subtract the Bad Additions

Some exponents of these leading diets say that caffeine has no place in healthful meals. Others say the same about excessive sodium. Some lambaste both. And when they all take aim against these dietary add-ons, they often shoot from completely different perspectives.

"We should do without caffeine," Szekely said. "Because caffeine is a stimulant, it can interrupt the messages of tiredness to the brain. People should know when they're truly tired, so they can do something about it."

"We suspect that caffeine interferes with prostaglandins [hormonelike regulators manufactured in the body]," Dr. Mannerberg says. "And we know for sure that it helps release stored fat into the bloodstream. For sedentary people, that can be downright dangerous."

And, as you know, excessive sodium intake has its own hazards. You've already heard that too much sodium in the diet—both from table salt and presalted foods—has been linked to high blood pressure, a major ingredient in the recipe for a heart attack. And that's precisely the view of the AHA. It's reflected in their diet and their call for general restraint with the saltshaker.

In the Pritikin diet, however, hypertension is not salt's chief evil—it's the edema, or fluid retention, that the salt causes. "The edema tends to deprive tissues of oxygen," he said, "thus creating a host of circulatory problems."

So in the Pritikin diet, sodium is restricted to about 2,000 milligrams a day, compared to the national average of 6,000 milligrams.

3. Get the Carbohydrates Right

Whole grains, vegetables, fruits—these are all high in complex carbohydrates, and they make up most of each of the five diets. While the average American diet contains about 46 percent carbohydrates, the Pritikin plan includes about 80 percent. Aerobic nutrition registers 63 percent. And the other three regimes generally give complex carbohydrates an unspecified majority.

On the other hand, the simple refined carbohydrates—sugar, honey, syrup and molasses—are roundly condemned. For good reason. They raise triglyceride levels, may increase fat and cholesterol in the blood and stress your pancreas.

For Dr. Mannerberg, a diet high in complex carbohydrates is an aerobic necessity. "They actually reduce serum triglyceride levels," he says. "And that can only be good news for your oxygen delivery system."

To Pritikin and Dr. Ornish, the supreme virtue of complex carbohydrates is their metabolic efficiency. Like simple carbohydrates, they convert into energy far better than protein or fat, leaving behind minimal waste. But unlike their simple, refined counterparts, they burn slowly, gingerly releasing glucose (the primary fuel for the brain) into the bloodstream, maintaining an even level of blood sugar.

All of which means that a diet packed with complex carbohydrates is reliable insurance against blood-sugar troubles. It's not surprising then that Pritikin reported success with his diet in treating hypoglycemics (people who suffer bouts of low blood sugar).

4. Balance Your Intake and Output

Implicit in most diets is the idea of the dietary balance sheet—your calorie intake versus your calorie use (physical exertion). When you take in more calories than you burn, you gain weight. When you burn more calories than you consume, you lose it. Every unburned 3,000 calories gathers to a pound of fat, and every ignited 3,000 means a pound lost. It's the old nutritional arithmetic, the doleful numbers game of the dieting life.

Advocates of our leading five, however, use new math. They still must reckon with the intake-output equation but find it easier to solve than most dieters do. That's because the diets emphasize complex carbohydrates, which are relatively low in calories. Eating a lot of them usually means losing weight, arriving quickly at a low balance point in the equation.

"When we put obese people on our high-carbohydrate diet," says Dr. Ornish, "they lost weight, even though they ate until they were satisfied. And when we tried the diet on people of normal weight, they maintained their weight."

Practitioners of the five regimes also work on the output side of the equation—they recommend exercise. Dr. Mannerberg talks about the Mannerberg method of movement, an exercise technique featuring constant motion. Szekely urges a similar mode of continuous exertion. And Pritikin extolled the joys of walking. They all acknowledge the medical facts: A side effect of increased output through exercise is better health.

5. Include Dietary Fiber

A diet big on complex carbohydrates is a diet big on fiber. But even if the two didn't go together, the advocates of our top-ranking diets would find a way to work fiber in.

Says Dr. Mannerberg, "Dr. Denis Burkitt and Dr. Hugh Trowell of England were the first medical investigators to make us aware of the problems associated with a low-fiber diet. They disclosed that many of the degenerative diseases in Western countries could correlate well with the amount of nutrient fiber in the diet."

Pritikin, Szekely, the AHA and thousands of vegetarians would surely nod in agreement, mentioning ulcers, diverticular disease, hemorrhoids and varicose veins among the problems that may be largely preventable with fiber.

And now you know the watchwords of some of the best diets in the land: low intake of fat, salt, sugar and caffeine; high intake of complex carbohydrates and fiber; and balanced caloric input and output. They represent the broad outlines of regimes that work, an invitation for you to fill in the fine print.

When you do work out the details, you may end up on middle ground, somewhere between the puritanic Pritikin regimen and the relatively lax AHA plan. And we think that's just where you should be. The Pritikin strictures would be difficult for most people to live with, and the AHA requirements simply don't go far enough. The Pritikin plan sets the fat level at 5 to 10 percent of caloric intake. The AHA suggests a 30 to 35 percent mark. We recommend the mid-range — 20 to 25 percent.

To get to that level you'd cut back on the fats implicitly sanctioned by the AHA. You'd halve that recommended intake of two to four tablespoons of polyunsaturated oil or margarine daily; avoid those cooking fats by doing more broiling, boiling and steaming; and try to stay clear of meats like pork or lamb. You'd also take a more moderate approach toward certain foods severely limited or banned outright by the Pritikin diet. You wouldn't blacklist nuts, seeds and fish, for they have too many redeeming nutritional qualities. And you wouldn't ban butter and margarine. You'd simply eat them sparingly.

CHAPTER 2

How to Lose 10 Pounds without Dieting or Jogging

Listen in, all you diehard dieters. Have we got news for you! There really *is* a secret to getting thin, and it has nothing to do with dieting.

It's not another one of those quick-weight-loss schemes (high protein, low protein, no protein . . .). Nor is there a gimmick. It's simply an easy, sensible way to lose weight naturally. And you don't have to give up your favorite foods or run around the track until you melt into butter, either.

Let's say you want to lose ten pounds. Now anybody who's ever been on a diet knows that one pound lost is equal to about 3,000 calories. If you just cut out or burn off 300 calories a day, you can lose about a pound every ten days. Cut back 500 calories a day, and you'll be able to lose about a pound a week.

All it takes is learning how to burn off those calories faster and more efficiently. But before any of this starts to make sense, you must first understand a few things about diets.

First off, they don't work. Anyone who keeps three different sizes of clothing in the closet can tell you that. Diets, in the words of Gabe Mirkin, M.D., are "anti-Nature."

"Studies have shown that the success rate of anyone going on a diet and keeping the weight off one year later is one in 10. After five years, it's one in 20," says the author of *Getting Thin* (Little, Brown and Company).

When it comes to dieting, the body's defenses often outweigh the mind's determination. "When caloric intake is reduced, the body does everything in its power to conserve energy," Dr. Mirkin says.

He explained that the body has an adaptive hormone called reverse T_3, which goes into action when calories are reduced. "This hormone slows down the metabolism. An average 150-pound person burns about 70 calories an hour while sleeping. When he's dieting, it's reduced to about 40 calories an hour and the process is slowed down all day long. It's the body's defense against starvation."

Second, there's the notion that just looking at food can make some people gain weight. That may sound ludicrous, but it's closer to the truth than you may think.

This was demonstrated at Yale University, where psychologist Judith Rodin, Ph.D., measured the reactions in a group of former fat people to a thick, juicy steak sizzling on a grill in front of them. It was to be their reward after an 18-hour fast. Dr. Rodin took blood samples as they watched the steak cooking.

"Those who were highly responsive to the steak cooking before them also had high levels of insulin release," Dr. Rodin says. "Being turned on just by the sight of food set their metabolic process in motion. Insulin accelerates the intake of fat into the cells, so the more insulin that is secreted the faster the fat will be stored."

In short, those who drooled over the steak turned more of it into fat than those who didn't.

"We think 60 to 70 percent of the people who are moderately overweight are like this," says Dr. Rodin.

Ever wonder why you keep returning to your original weight, time and time again, no matter how you struggle? That's where diet-blocker number three comes in. It's known as the set-point theory.

The body has a control system—sort of an inner thermostat for body fat—that seeks a constant set amount of fat in the body. It's the weight you're unthinkingly drawn to, give or take a few pounds, say William Bennett, M.D., and Joel Gurin in their book *The Dieter's Dilemma* (Basic Books). Fatties have high set points and string beans have low set points. It's as simple as that.

Ugh! Sounds discouraging, doesn't it?

Now you'll be better able to understand why exercise is so important. Just a moderate amount of exercise can help speed up your metabolism, lower your set point and even reduce your craving for food. As little as a half-hour walk is good for 100 to 150 calories—up to half of your 300-calorie-a-day goal. Walk twice a day and you'll be well on your way to the 500-calorie-a-day mark. The rest will come by changing your eating habits. But we'll get to that later.

Routine exercise can boost a dieter's sluggish 40-calorie-an-hour metabolic rate to 70 or 80 calories an hour, says Dr. Mirkin. "Just a half hour a day will keep you burning calories at a faster rate all day long.

"Many people are discouraged from exercising when they find out that in order to lose a single pound they must run for four hours, ice-skate nine hours, play volleyball 10 hours or walk 17 hours," he says. "But you don't need to do all that exercise at one time. If you spread those hours over a week or two, you'll have lost a substantial amount of weight by the end of the year."

But, as we said in the beginning, you don't have to jog or do other strenuous exercise. Walking can help you lose weight, too. This was proved several years back by a group of obese women in California who lost an average of 22 pounds each in one year simply by adding a walk to their daily routine.

Put Exercise on Your Menu

Participate in half an hour or more of moderate activity daily and you'll be well on your way to permanent weight loss. The list below can give you an idea of the calories that can be expended during these common activities.

Moderate Activity	Calories per Hour*
Walking (2½ mph)	210
Walking (3¾ mph)	300
Bicycling (5½ mph)	210
Gardening	220
Golf	250
Bowling	270
Swimming (¼ mph)	300
Square dancing	350
Volleyball	350
Roller skating	350

---

*Energy expenditure by a 150-pound person.

All 11 women in the experiment were chronic dieters who were never successful at keeping off any of the weight they had lost on repeated calorie-cutting regimens. This time there were no dietary restrictions, but a daily walk was a must. Weight loss didn't start until walks routinely exceeded 30 minutes a day. When weight stabilized, walking time was increased and weight loss resumed.

The importance of walking was demonstrated even better by two women in the group who started to regain weight after they became ill and stopped exercising. But once walking resumed, weight loss started all over again (*Archives of Internal Medicine,* May, 1975).

Now, of course, comes the excuse that exercise only makes you want to eat more. Not so, say the experts.

Scientists found this out by counting the calories consumed by a group of obese women who were allowed to eat all they wanted during the two-month experiment.

Each underwent three 19-day treatments—one sedentary period, a period of mild daily treadmill exercise and a period of moderate treadmill exercise. Although they gradually became more active, their caloric intake did not increase (*American Journal of Clinical Nutrition,* September, 1982).

Enough said about exercise. Now we come to the other daily 200 or 300 calories you want to avoid at meals to reach your ten-pound goal. Psychologists have dubbed the approach "behavior modification." It means you've got to adopt a whole new way of looking at food—and swallowing it, too.

Say Goodbye to the Binge

"Overweight is simply a matter of food abuse," says Laura Jane Walker, Ph.D., a weight-control specialist in Los Angeles. "People like to blame it on boredom, but that's just an excuse. Overweight people in general have a pattern of anger, eat, anger, eat." It's a malady known as a "binge."

"Many people grab a piece of pizza, look at it as fattening, say 'I blew the diet' and continue stuffing themselves with pizza," says Dr. Walker. "What's needed here is a behavior change."

Dr. Walker believes that such a person could be thoroughly satisfied with just one slice of the pizza by taking smaller bites and eating it slowly.

"In my classes I make people take a piece of food and really chew it for as long as possible," she says. "I tell them to chew it slowly, to roll it around the mouth and savor the flavor. For the first time, some of them actually *taste* the food. People who wolf down food never taste it. Getting pleasure out of tasting will satisfy you with less.

Dr. Walker also recommends stretching a meal out as long as possible, at least 20 minutes—the amount of time it takes the brain to tell the stomach the hunger is gone. "Eating slowly improves assimilation of nutrients," says Dr. Walker. "Digestion is improved many times over."

Eating most of your calories early in the day is another way to promote weight loss. In one study, seven volunteers ate 2,000 calories a day at breakfast and all seven lost weight. But when they ate the same 2,000 calories as an evening meal, they lost less weight, or even *gained* weight. Dieters, say the scientists who conducted the study, should consider "the importance of timing apart from the amount of caloric intake" (*Chronobiologia,* vol. 3, no. 1, 1976).

Eat Light at Night

One reason for this is that digestion doesn't peak until about seven hours after the last swallow. If most of the calories were eaten at the evening meal, digestion time comes around while you're sleeping, the time when your metabolism is at its lowest ebb.

"People on a normal 9-to-5 schedule should take all their meals before 7 P.M.," says Dr. Walker, who has lost and successfully kept off 30 pounds through behavior modification.

She also recommends eating most of your protein at lunch rather than dinner. "That way you'll be burning the protein when you're the most active."

Eating smaller, frequent meals rather than a few large meals is another good habit to adopt. For one thing, "skipping meals makes you famished and you'll want to attack the food when the next meal rolls around," says Dr. Walker.

A way to beat hunger pangs is practiced widely in Beverly Hills by the patients of Arnold Fox, M.D. He recommends carrying around a bag of vegetables for constant munching throughout the day.

Carbohydrates Are Important

"Eating vegetables makes you feel satisfied and full. Not only that, you're not as hungry when mealtime rolls around," Dr. Fox says. "If you're going to a party or out to dinner, eat an apple or a few carrots before you leave the house. You'll be surprised at how many calories you can save that way."

Fresh vegetables come under the label of complex carbohydrates, which is another key to losing weight with ease. Complex carbohydrates are healthful because of their effect on the release of glucose in the bloodstream. They work to release glucose slowly and over a longer period of time, keeping blood sugar on an even keel. "Complex carbohydrates are also high in fiber, which helps speed up food passage through the system—another aid in losing weight," says Dr. Fox.

Complex carbohydrates should not be confused with simple carbohydrates. The complex variety are found in foods such as starchy vegetables, whole grains and brown rice. Simple carbohydrates are represented by refined sugars and tabletop syrups.

Adding soup to your diet can also lower your caloric intake. The most recent study was conducted by a team of researchers including Jack Smith, Ph.D., director of medical nutrition education at the University of Nebraska Medical Center and the Swanson Center for Nutrition. They analyzed the dietary records of 28,000 individuals, and found that those who ate soup consumed roughly 5 percent fewer calories than those who didn't. "And that counts for all age groups," says Dr. Smith.

Dr. Smith sees several reasons why soup can be beneficial as a reducing aid. "One thing is that soup contains a lot of water, so it's not calorically dense. Also, soup is generally made out of vegetables, so there aren't many calories there, either. It's hot, so you eat it slower, making it easier to stretch the meal out to 20 minutes."

Soup and complex carbohydrates—they're proven weight-loss aids that can put you well on your way to your goal. But that's not all. Our experts have passed on some other practical tips and tricks:

• Drink plenty of water—up to eight glasses a day. It fills you up and there are no calories. Just remember that most foods are more than 50 percent water. So, when you feel hungry, ask yourself: "Could it be a glass of water that I want?"

• Take up a project, one that keeps your hands busy or even dirty so you'll find it impossible to reach for food when monotony hits. Dr. Rodin says she's found this helps food lovers keep their minds off snacking. "Make sure you're busy at the time of the day you're most tempted by food," she suggests. "If you get caught up in the project, you won't even think about food."

• Put your meals on luncheon plates rather than dinner plates. It gives you the illusion of eating more when you're really not.

• Always sit at the table, and never read or watch television while eating. It only distracts you and can make you eat more than you really want or need.

• Eat vegetarian meals at least one day a week. You'll almost always eat fewer calories and take in less fat. You'll load up on nutrients, too.

• Put down your knife and fork or sandwich between bites. You'll be surprised how much longer your meal will last.

• Cut down on salad dressing by mixing the salad and dressing in a large bowl first rather than putting a dollop on top of the greens at the dinner table. Remember that one tablespoon of salad dressing contains 80 calories. A little can go a long way if it is mixed correctly.

• Always cut the skin away from chicken, before cooking, if possible. The skin is high in fat and adds calories you can easily do without. Ditto with fat on steaks and chops.

• Break the fried-food habit. Always choose a baked potato instead of french fries, or broiled fish rather than deep fried.

• Don't pour gravy all over your food. Instead put it on the side and dip a corner of the food into it. You'll consume a lot less for the same flavor.

• Gradually cut down your consumption of red meat and eat more fish and fowl. You'll save calories, help lower your cholesterol and improve your overall health.

• Get a coach. Let a friend or family member in on what you're trying to do. Make sure it's someone who cares—someone who can smack your wrist when you go astray and pat you on the back for a job well done.

• Never eat when you're not hungry.

So forget the fat farms, weight belts and rubberized suits. Throw out the diet pills.

Remember that getting thin can be your reward for good food sense at the dinner table. Simply follow the rules of good behavior and chances are slim that you'll ever get fat again.

CHAPTER 3

Perk Up Your Metabolism and Peel Off Pounds

If you're overweight, you know it's no small injustice. Your reed-slim friend can win a pie-eating contest and not gain an ounce. You on the other hand seem to put on five pounds just thinking about pie.

You have a sneaking suspicion that your metabolism is out of whack, but you don't dare suggest it. Most medical experts regard "It's my metabolism" as a lame cover-up for all those second helpings you obviously indulged in and the chocolate bars they're sure you've stashed in the glove compartment of your car.

But these days they're not so quick to prescribe a diet and a dose of guilt. It truly may not be your fault. Recent studies, still controversial, indicate that all metabolisms are not created equal. Your skinny pie-eating friend may have a metabolism that allows her to burn up all those excess calories as heat while yours stores them as fat.

Don't be alarmed, though. You're not doomed. There's evidence you can get your metabolism revved up by new patterns and combinations of exercise, diet and everyday habits. Why change your ways? To take advantage of a still mysterious metabolic phenomenon called dietary-induced thermogenesis.

Though quite a mouthful, it simply means that your body generates heat after you've eaten. That's why you often push away from a large meal feeling uncomfortably warm. You can get that same feeling after vigorous exercise, and, of course, that's no coincidence. Something similar is happening.

When you exercise, your body is burning up calories. The digestive process is a calorie-burning activity, too. After a meal the body works hard to store what you've eaten as fuel. Though it retains some food energy as fat, it gives off some as heat. And the more you burn off as heat, the less you store as fat.

Some of the latest research has shown that overweight people many times do not eat more than their thinner counterparts. They simply have sluggish metabolisms that don't generate that slimming after-dinner blaze. And dieting doesn't help. Their efficient, fat-storing metabolisms regard even a moderate caloric cutback as a signal that starvation is at hand and begin to store fat in case the food shortage goes on indefinitely.

But here's the real news. Exercise can fan the flames of even a "sluggish" metabolism—in at least four different ways. The *timing* of your meals and your exercise can also help your slimming program.

Peter M. Miller, Ph.D., director of the Hilton Head Health Institute, Hilton Head, South Carolina, teaches his clients to pare the pounds off by fanning those fires. The double whammy of *The Hilton Head Metabolism Diet* (Warner Books) is a low-calorie but four-meal-a-day diet and moderate but well-timed exercise.

The aim of the Hilton Head Diet is to get those fires stoked and keep them burning all day long. Dr. Miller says he divided his low-calorie diet into four meals to take advantage of the after-meal thermic effect. After all, digestion burns up calories. And before the blaze becomes a pile of embers, Dr. Miller recommends a brisk 20-minute walk. If done no later than 20 minutes after at least two meals a day, your postmeal heat production can be enhanced by up to 50 percent, he says. So, if your digestive processes normally burn 100 calories, a brisk walk for 20 minutes could increase that to 150. Do that after two meals each day and that's 36,500 calories a year—more than 10 pounds of fat." Exercise after meals burns calories more efficiently than any other exercise schedule," Dr. Miller says. "It's at this time that you're primed to increase your metabolic rate. So, step on the gas. Take advantage of this maximum time."

Once you master two brisk walks a day, you might want to consider graduating into more aerobic exercises. Researchers at the University of New Hampshire found that an increase in aerobic capacity (your body's ability to use oxygen) significantly increases the number of calories you burn after a meal—even if you're *not* exercising at that particular time.

16

When they tested dietary-induced thermogenesis in a group of men and women, they discovered that those with greater aerobic capacity burned more calories after eating (or, in this case, drinking high- and low-calorie drinks). And the men (but not the women) were more likely to have a lower percentage of body fat. The best news, however, is that those not terribly fit people who improved their aerobic capacity by exercise were *also* able to stoke their after-meal blaze. One woman who increased her aerobic capacity by only 15 percent boosted her heat response by 110 percent (*European Journal of Applied Physiology,* vol. 50, no. 3, 1983).

Not everyone is going to be able to achieve the aerobic fitness of a well-conditioned athlete. Many of them have metabolisms that allow them to burn hundreds of calories doing nothing more strenuous than watching television. Aerobic capacity can be increased only within limits because it largely depends on the number of muscle fibers you're born with. But, though you can't add muscle fibers, you can make the ones you have more effective through aerobic exercise.

Jogging, tennis, dancing—anything that gets your heart pumping and your muscles moving and forces your body to break down fat for energy—can increase your aerobic capacity. Aerobic exercise for 30 minutes three times a week will stimulate your metabolism so that you'll burn calories at a faster rate than usual for as long as 24 hours after exercise—*in addition* to the hundreds you'll be burning during the exercise. "Aerobic activity stimulates the metabolism better than any other factor," says Dr. Miller.

It does something else, too. It increases your muscle mass at the same time it reduces the amount of fat you're carrying. People who have a high ratio of muscle to fat have higher metabolic rates. They can eat more and not gain weight because they burn more, even when they're sleeping.

"The reason for this is that muscle tissue is metabolically more active than fat tissue," Dr. Miller says. "It takes more body energy for muscle to function. Fat is relatively inactive, while muscle cells are extremely active, even when you are resting. A muscle furnace is constantly burning food fuel at a rapid rate day after day."

So to review, exercise can boost your metabolism in at least three different ways—in addition to the immediate calorie burnoff. First, when exercise follows a meal, it increases dietary thermogenesis— "roasting" calories that would otherwise be stored as fat. Second, regular aerobic exercise increases metabolism all day long—giving an extra boost after meals even if you're just reading a book. And third, by adding muscle, with its high metabolic rate, you're subtracting extra calories from your system every moment of the day.

But exercise and meal timing aren't the only factors that affect your metabolism. What you eat, even the temperature of your home, can either fan the fires or hose them down.

Food Choices

Eat more fruits, vegetables and whole grains, the complex carbohydrates. Avoid fats and simple carbohydrates (candy, soft drinks, desserts). Elliot Danforth Jr., M.D., director of the clinical research center at the University of Vermont, says a return "to the diet of our ancestors" can have a significant impact on obesity. That means a diet that is about two-thirds complex carbohydrates and the rest protein and fat. Why? "There's a clean biochemical reason for this," says Dr. Danforth, who did many of the early studies on metabolism and obesity. "You expend only about 3 percent of your fat calories storing them as fat, but you expend 25 percent of your carbohydrate calories storing them as fat. The metabolic cost is far higher to store carbohydrates as fat. Any Iowa pig farmer will tell you. When you ask him how he gets his pigs so fat, he'll tell you it isn't by feeding them wheat, it's by feeding them fat."

Climate

Extremes of heat or cold increase your metabolism by as much as 10 percent, says Dr. Miller. Even a small deviation helps. Set your thermostat at 68°F in the winter and 79°F in the summer. You'll get used to the temperatures and your metabolism will get a boost.

Like most sensible weight-loss regimens, this is a lifetime proposition. Once you perk up your metabolism, it will be your ally. But you've got to keep it perked up through diet and exercise.

CHAPTER 4

Best and Worst Diet Ideas

Diet Plan

BEST: *The Complete University Medical Diet,* detailed in the book by that name. An eminently intelligent approach that incorporates all the latest findings of science, as well as the experience of the author's weight-control program at Johns Hopkins University. Maria Simonson, Ph.D., who once weighed over 300 pounds and is now less than half that size, offers fascinating scientific revelations about overweight along with a host of practical tips and coping strategies. Published by Rawson Associates.

PERENNIAL FAVORITE: *Weight Watchers.* Many people find the help of a real live support group, in this or similar programs, more effective than even the best book.

STRANGEST: *The Blackmail Diet,* described in the book by that name, by John Bear, Ph.D. Dr. Bear asserts that most people won't stick to a reducing plan, no matter how good it is. His personal solution: "On Day 1, I put $5,000 into a binding, unbreakable trust. The terms of the trust were as follows: If I lost 75 pounds in the next 365 days, I got all my money back. If I failed to do so, the trustee was to turn the entire sum of money over to the American Nazi Party." It worked, he says!

And to make sure he didn't gain the weight back? Simple. "I've signed an agreement with my publisher. If I gain weight, all my royalties from the sale of this book go immediately to the Ku Klux Klan.

"I have successfully blackmailed myself," Dr. Bear gloats. "The same methods can work for everyone." Published by Ten Speed Press.
PHONIEST: *The Mayo Clinic Diet.* Ads for it appear regularly in magazines and newspapers, yet it has no connection whatsoever with the famous medical center. Doctors at the Rochester, Minnesota, institution told us the "diet" has been popping up for years, and they've never been able to eradicate it.
WORST: Any diet based on taking pills instead of changing lifestyle habits.

Signs of the Times

BEST: Sharing a dessert, going to the gym at lunch, not putting bread on the table.
WORST: Pizza shops that deliver, chocolate yogurt, soft drinks in cartons the size of wastebaskets.

Overheard Remarks

BEST: "We always made too much, so we just cook smaller portions now. . . . A big dessert makes me sleepy. . . . I know one cookie won't hurt, but I'm just not hungry."
WORST: "Don't you like my cooking? . . . Start your diet tomorrow! . . . Are you going to leave that good food on your plate?"

Thing to Skip

BEST: The second glass of wine or cocktail before dinner. That's the one that makes your mouth hyperactive—in more ways than one.
WORST: Breakfast. Jackie Storm, nutritionist at the New York Health & Racquet Club, says many of her clients with weight problems have a history of skipping breakfast. She gets them to eat *anything* for breakfast, then guides them into quality foods, like whole grain cereals or muffins. Can work wonders, says Jackie, by preventing uncontrolled eating at night.

Tricks of Mother Nature

BEST: Substantially overweight women (perhaps men, too) who begin exercising do not eat more food to compensate for the caloric expenditure. Normal-weight people do eat more, keeping their size stable.
WORST: Once the substantially overweight person has reduced, he or she—to stay at the new, lower weight—must often either exercise more or eat less than a person the same size who was never fat.

Simple Trick

BEST: Walk for 30 minutes—away from your house. Somehow, finding the motivation to walk the second 30 minutes is easy. Repeat once a day and you'll lose up to 30 or 40 pounds in a year—without dieting.
WORST: Black spandex clothing.

Way to "Melt Fat"

BEST: Going for a walk after you eat. Brings on "exercise-induced postprandial thermogenesis," which means the production of extra body heat created by exercising on a full stomach. This heat does in a real sense melt fat.
WORST: Taking any kind of pill. The only thing that will melt is your morale, when you discover it doesn't work.

Personal Resource

BEST: Time. Yes, time. If you can give yourself the gift of an hour a day to exercise—just walking is perfect—most of your problem is over. If you are the generous sort, give yourself an hour and a half a day during the week, two hours or more during weekends.
WORST: Willpower.

Substitution

BEST: Herb or malt vinegar on fish and vegetables instead of tartar sauce or butter. A fresh new taste that can easily save 100 calories per meal.
WORST: A croissant instead of buttered toast. Starts your day with 130 extra calories.

Indulgence

BEST: A week at a health spa.
WORST: A cushy reclining chair and nearby remote TV control. Suitable for fracture patients, risky for others.

Auspicious Combination of Letters

BEST: Words beginning with N-O, as in no more, not for me, no thank you, and now or never.
WORST: Words beginning with M-A as in marzipan, Mallomars, marmalade, mayonnaise, madeleines, Mars bars, macadamia nuts and marble cake.

21

Place to Spend a Day

BEST: Yosemite or any other national park where walking is a thrill, and you discover the joys of fitness and serenity.
WORST: Solvang, California, a tourist town whose main industry is Danish-pastry shops.

Fitness Equipment

BEST: Good walking or running shoes.
WORST: Anything that can be used only while lying down.

Child-Rearing Idea

BEST: The notion that a child's eating habits require just as much firm, loving discipline as homework or cleanliness.
WORST: That children must clean their plates.

Inventions of the Future

BEST: Electronic label scanners at supermarket checkouts that tally not only prices, but the nutritional value of your purchases.
WORST: Chocolate-Covered Macadamia Nut "Gourmet" Ice Cream packaged in two-gallon troughs.

Shape to Strive For

BEST: Any shape at all that would cause a child, asked to pick out "the fat one" from a group of five people, to ignore you.
WORST: Having not a visible ounce of fat on your body, not one sag or crease or dimple. Take a good look at the statues of the Greek goddesses or Olympic gold medal gymnast Mary Lou Retton, and you'll notice even they aren't thin enough for modern worshippers of sainthood-by-skinniness. Today's epidemic of harmful crash dieting, pill taking, anorexia and bulimia is directly traceable to the worship of this unrealistic and pointless ideal. Isn't it time for a second coming of Common Sense?

Dining-Out Development

BEST: "Spa Cuisine" at the elegant Four Seasons in New York. Low-fat, low-calorie, full of fresh taste and nutrition. The cold bass salad, for instance, offers a fillet of striped bass cooked with saffron and jalapeño peppers, and it's served with cool slices of mango and papaya, four different greens, mushrooms, radish sprouts and herb sauce.
WORST: The bass costs $33.

22

Fine-Dining Advice

Here, both sides of the street are covered by Andrew Birsh, editor and publisher of the *Restaurant Reporter* (71 Vanderbilt Ave., Room 320P, New York, NY 10169). In this gem of a newsletter, Birsh and staff detail their dining experiences in some of the most exciting and—potentially—most fattening restaurants in New York City. Yet, Birsh told us, "Eating out needn't harm you. There are slim and healthy people in the best restaurants." So, here is the voice of experience:

Overall Strategy

BEST: The goal is to have a good time eating. And part of that is to leave feeling good, which usually means not eating everything in sight. Most restaurants bloat up the meal for the eye, not the stomach. Don't feel you have to eat the whole thing—eat the amount that is right for you.

As reviewers, we sample; we don't wolf down the whole thing. I follow the "hemisphere diet": I divide the plate in half and eat only from half of the plate.

WORST: Going to a buffet or smorgasbord. Unless you have a will of iron, it's trouble.

Ethnic Restaurants

BEST: Chinese or Japanese. Light food, the least fat, more vegetables. High-quality carbohydrates.

WORST: Eastern European, Hungarian, German, some kinds of English food, very refined French restaurants.

WORST YET: Eating fried foods in a bar, with beer and snacks off the counter. Full of empty calories.

What to Order at a Good Restaurant

BEST: You're in luck if you like fish. Ask for it to be cooked simply. Ask for sauce on the side. Often restaurants balk at not giving sauce, but sauce on the side they'll do. Salads with dressing on the side. Watch out for dessert. Many restaurants have fresh fruit desserts; they can be served elegantly. Ask for cream or custard sauce on the side.

WORST: Surf & turf—a disaster with high fat and high calories.

CHAPTER 5

Lighten Up!

Joan's been trying to lose those extra ten pounds for years. Sure, she diets for a couple of weeks, but when she gets to the point where she can't face one more celery stalk or turn down one more dessert, it's back to bingeing. She knows heavy isn't healthy, but dieting's just too difficult.

John's just found out that he has high blood pressure. His doctor told him to cut down the amount of sodium in his diet, but he didn't tell him how. When John began reading the labels on the foods he usually eats, he was shocked at the high sodium content. And because John works late most evenings, he doesn't always have time to prepare his own no-salt, made-from-scratch meals. Now he's ready to give up.

Enter "lite" foods. Because they're lower in salt, calories, sugar or cholesterol than the regular versions, these tasty new products can help people like Joan and John achieve their goals.

"Lite foods have great potential to help people lose weight," says Kelly D. Brownell, Ph.D., co-director of the Obesity Research Clinic at the University of Pennsylvania School of Medicine. "But there are still several questions. Can they constitute enough of the total calorie intake to have an impact on weight, and are they acceptable to dieters?"

The answer to both questions, we've found, is a resounding yes! In a preliminary study by the Health, Weight and Stress Program at the Johns Hopkins Medical Institutions, researchers found that lite foods really did help people lose weight.

The researchers worked with over 100 overweight people and divided them into two groups. One group followed a standard low-calorie reducing diet. The other group, however, was asked to cut calories by eating lite foods. Over a four-month period, the people who ate lite foods each lost five to seven pounds *more* than the people on the standard reduction diet.

Staying Motivated

According to Maria Simonson, Ph.D., Sc.D., director of the program and co-author of *The Complete University Medical Diet* (Rawson Associates), the dieters found the lite foods not only acceptable but downright appealing. "The psychological effect was marvelous! These foods helped people maintain a nutritionally balanced, low-calorie diet without the usual feelings of boredom or deprivation. They stayed very motivated."

"If you feel better about a diet, you'll stick with it," says Janet Gailey-Phipps, Ph.D., another researcher on the study. "We actually found that people really liked the lite foods. After all, if you love certain foods, you have to be able to have them once in a while. Take desserts, for instance. People don't feel like giving them up forever. We found that the people in our study especially liked the lite desserts."

But it takes more than just low-calorie desserts to make a diet work. Luckily, variety is the spice of lite. In fact, there are so many different lite foods on the market nowadays, from frozen entrees to no-longer-forbidden fruit, that for the first time dieters can have real variety. And according to Dr. Gailey-Phipps, that's very important. "The successful dieters in our study used a wide variety of lite food products, including fruit, cheese, margarine, bread, soup and even beer! As long as you still consider the total calories eaten each day and keep to your diet plan, lite foods can be an extra added attraction of your weight-loss program."

In another current study, researchers are using lite foods to help fight high blood pressure. The Hypertension Prevention Trial, funded by the National Institutes of Health, is a national study being conducted at four major universities. The study is trying to prevent high blood pressure in people who are at high risk by changing their diets. The participants are encouraged to reduce their salt intake and to lose weight, if necessary. That's where lite foods come in.

"We find the new lite salad dressings to be extremely helpful," says Karen Levine, M.S., R.D., of the University of Mississippi Medical Center, nutritionist for the study. "Many people cut calories by eating a salad instead of a heavier meal, but if they drown it in high-calorie dressing, it's self-defeating." And if the dressing is high in sodium, it's double trouble.

A Little Lite Reading

Just because a package sports the words "lite" or "light" doesn't necessarily mean the food inside is low calorie. In fact, we found one brand of snack chips labeled "lights" that had exactly the same number of calories as the regular chips. So dieter beware! You still must read labels carefully.

Here are some pointers to guide you through the aisles:

- If it says "low calorie" on the label, the food contains no more than 40 calories per serving.
- "Reduced calorie" means that the food is at least one-third lower in calories than the regular kind.
- If a label indicates that calories have been cut, it must back it up with numbers comparing the reduced-calorie food with the unmodified version.
- A food labeled "sugar-free" or "sugarless" might not be low in calories. If that's the case, the label must say so.

The following Food and Drug Administration sodium-labeling rules took effect in July, 1985:

- If the label says "low-sodium," the product contains no more than 140 milligrams of sodium in each serving.
- "Very low sodium" denotes a product with 35 milligrams of sodium or less per serving.
- A "sodium-free" product has less than 5 milligrams per serving.
- To be called "reduced sodium," the normal level of sodium in a product must be reduced by 75 percent.
- "Unsalted" means that a food was made without salt when salt is normally used in processing.

"We take a look at each person's eating pattern and substitute low-sodium versions of the foods they already use," says Ms. Levine. "We're having a lot of success with that approach. When dietary changes are too drastic, people revert to their old eating habits pretty quickly."

The most useful lite items are those that replace foods we rely on heavily. For example, if someone uses margarine frequently, switching to the unsalted kind can cut a lot of sodium out of his or her diet. And because they're used in so many dishes, unsalted canned tomato products are an area ripe for ridding ourselves of extra salt.

Lite foods *are* helping people keep their weight and blood pressure down. But what if you don't have high blood pressure or a weight problem?

You too can benefit from lite eating. For one thing, turning on to lite foods can help you protect your heart. The American Heart Association recommends that people control their intake of cholesterol. And evidence shows that most Americans eat more sodium and fat than they need. Sugar, too, is a bad guy we'd all be better off avoiding.

The fact is, there are lots of reasons to eat lite. And with the abundance of streamlined products available now, healthier eating and a slimmer waist are almost a cinch.

Deliciously Lite Recipes

Peachy Sprout Salad

2 cups bean sprouts
1 16-ounce can lite peaches, drained and cubed
1 cup shredded carrots
¼ cup raisins

1 tablespoon lemon juice
2 tablespoons lite mayonnaise
2 tablespoons low-fat yogurt
1 teaspoon vanilla

In a medium-size mixing bowl, toss together the bean sprouts, peaches, carrots and raisins. In a cup, combine the lemon juice, mayonnaise, yogurt and vanilla. Spoon the dressing over the salad and toss to combine. Serves 4 to 6.

Potato-Cheese Dream

2 large potatoes, cooked and cut into ¼-inch slices	2 eggs
	1 cup low-fat cottage cheese
1 cup shredded lite cheese	pinch of cayenne pepper
2 scallions, chopped	¼ cup minced fresh parsley

In an oiled 8 × 8-inch baking dish, layer ½ of the potatoes, then ½ of the cheese, then ½ of the scallions. Repeat the sequence. Blend together the eggs and cottage cheese in a food processor or blender. Stir in the cayenne and ½ of the parsley.

Pour this sauce over the potatoes, cheese and onions. Sprinkle the remaining parsley on top. Bake at 375°F for 20 to 30 minutes, or until the top is lightly browned. Serves 6.

Lima Bean Cheese Loaf

2 cups cooked lima beans	¼ cup minced onions
1 cup skim milk	¼ teaspon garlic powder
1 cup whole wheat bread crumbs	3 eggs, beaten
1½ cups shredded lite cheese	1 cup no-salt tomato sauce, heated

Combine the lima beans and milk in a blender or food processor and puree. Combine the bread crumbs, cheese, onions, and garlic powder in a medium-size mixing bowl. Stir in the lima bean puree, then mix in the eggs.

Turn into a greased 8 × 4-inch loaf pan. Place the loaf pan in a larger pan and add 1 inch of hot water. Bake at 350°F for 1 hour or until a knife inserted in the center comes out clean. Serve with the hot tomato sauce. Serves 6.

Apple Custard Pudding

1 cup lite applesauce	1 tablespoon vanilla
3 eggs	¼ teaspoon nutmeg
½ cup skim milk	2 tablespoons raisins
1-2 tablespoons honey	
grated rind and juice of	
½ lemon	

Beat together all of the ingredients in a medium-size mixing bowl. Pour into a buttered 1½-quart casserole. Place the casserole inside a larger shallow baking pan. Add enough hot water to the pan to reach about halfway up the sides of the casserole. Bake at 350°F for 50 minutes or until a knife inserted in the center comes out clean. Chill before serving. Serves 4.

Lite Cheese Soufflé

This soufflé is extra-lite because it's made without butter.

3 tablespoons whole wheat flour	1 cup shredded lite cheese
1 cup milk	4 eggs, separated

Preheat the oven to 400°F.

In a medium-size saucepan, beat the flour and milk together until well blended. Cook over medium heat, stirring constantly with a wire whisk, until thickened. Reduce heat and whisk in the cheese. Continue stirring until melted. Beat the egg yolks in a cup, whisk into the cheese mixture, and cook, stirring constantly, for another minute. Let cool slightly.

In a medium-size bowl, beat the egg whites until very stiff. Blend ¼ of the egg whites with the cheese mixture. Gently fold in the remaining egg whites.

Turn into a lightly oiled 1½-quart soufflé dish. Place in the oven. Turn the heat down to 350°F and bake for 30 to 35 minutes. Serves 4 to 6.

Yogurt Chicken Paprika

2 onions, thinly sliced
2 tablepoons lite margarine
1 3-pound chicken, cut into
    serving pieces and
    skinned, if desired

1 tablespoon paprika
⅓ cup chicken stock
1 cup low-fat yogurt

Sauté the onions in the margarine in a large, heavy skillet until golden. Move the onions to the side of the pan, add the chicken pieces, and fry until lightly browned, about 10 minutes.

Reduce heat to low, arrange the chicken skin-side up, sprinkle with the paprika and add the stock. Cover and simmer for 45 minutes or until the chicken is tender.

Remove the chicken and keep warm. Mix the yogurt into the sauce and heat briefly. Do not boil. Pour the sauce over the chicken. Serves 4.

Spanish Rice

1 large onion, minced
1 clove garlic, minced
1 tablespoon lite margarine
1 small green pepper, minced
½ cup brown rice

½ teaspoon chili powder
1 16-ounce can no-salt
    tomatoes
½ cup water
1 bay leaf

Sauté the onions and garlic in the margarine in a large saucepan until the onions are soft. Add the green peppers and sauté for 4 to 5 minutes more. Stir in the rice and chili powder and sauté for another minute. Add the tomatoes, including the juice, along with the water and bay leaf. Stir briefly, crushing the tomatoes slightly. Cover and simmer for 40 to 45 minutes. Remove the bay leaf. Serves 4.

Baked Pears with Almonds

1 28-ounce can lite pears,
    drained and cut into
    ¼-inch slices
¼ cup maple syrup
1 teaspoon vanilla

½ cup sliced almonds
¼ cup wheat germ
2 tablespoons lite margarine,
    melted

Layer the pears in an oiled 8 × 8-inch baking dish. In a cup, combine the syrup and vanilla and drizzle over the pears. Sprinkle with the almonds and wheat germ. Drizzle the margarine on top. Bake at 350°F for 10 minutes or until hot, basting occasionally. Serves 6.

The Lite Stuff

Are you in the dark about lite foods? To help you see just what you're getting, or *not* getting, we've compared some representative products with their lite substitutes.

Food	Portion	Regular	Lite
		Calories	
Breaded fish fillets	6 oz.	300	276
Fruited yogurt	1 cup	260	240
Cottage cheese	½ cup	130	90
Monterey Jack cheese	1 oz.	110	50
Applesauce	4 oz.	105	50
Mayonnaise	1 tbsp.	101	40
Pancake syrup	2 tbsp.	100	50
Fruit cocktail	½ cup	97	50
		Sodium (mg.)	
Tomato sauce	4 oz.	665	25
Vegetable juice cocktail	6 oz.	555	60
Tomato juice	6 oz.	550	20
American cheese	1 oz.	406	89
Tuna	3 oz.	338	180
Ketchup	1 tbsp.	169	6
Muenster cheese	1 oz.	132	10
Butter	1 tbsp.	115	2
Stoned wheat crackers	5	95	2
French dressing	1 tbsp.	20	5
		Cholesterol (mg.)	
Eggs	1 large	240	0
Cheddar cheese	1 oz.	30	10

CHAPTER 6

Drink Up and
Slim Down

Which has more calories: a nut-filled brownie or an accompanying glass of milk; a mug of beer or a whiskey sour; a glass of orange juice or a glass of Coca-Cola?

If you don't have a clue, it's probably because you're not used to thinking about the calorie content of beverages. After all, solid food is where most of the world's calories lurk right? Serious weight watchers fret about the fattening possibilities of gingerbread cakes, pumpkin pies and oversized eclairs. But who cares about liquid calories?

Maybe we all should. For some people, beverages may account for close to 50 percent of total calorie intake. For most of us the percentage is probably far higher than we think. And there are scores of drinks with higher calorie counts than any of the above sinfully caloric desserts. Besides, it's easier to substitute a low-calorie beverage for a high-calorie one if you know where all the calories are hiding.

Lesson number one: A glass of whole milk packs 159 calories but a brownie only 97; a mug of regular beer has about 150 calories but a whiskey sour 184; and a glass of orange juice carries 84 calories but a glass of Coke 72.

You'll find more surprises here in the accompanying liquid calorie guide, possibly the largest calorie counter for beverages ever assembled.

Our information comes from government nutrition data banks, manufacturers, and in some cases, from laboratory analyses.

Here's to a wiser and slimmer you!

Beverage Caloric Guide

Fruit Juices

Beverage	Serving Size (fl. oz.)	Calories per Serving	Calories per Ounce
Apple cider	8	118	15
Apple juice	8	118	15
Knudsen cherry cider	8	96	12
Apricot nectar	7	125	18
Pear nectar	5½	100	18
Libby's peach nectar	6	90	15
Guava nectar	6	300	50
Knudsen papaya nectar	8	104	13
Cranapple juice, regular	8	173	22
Cranapple juice, low-calorie	8	43	5
Cranberry juice cocktail, regular	8	141	18
Cranberry juice cocktail, low-calorie	8	48	6
Crangrape juice	8	144	18
Cranprune juice	8	154	19
Prune juice	2	45	23
Grape juice	8	170	21
Grapefruit juice, fresh	8	96	12
Grapefruit juice, canned	8	101	13
Knudsen pink grapefruit juice	8	76	10
Limeade, from frozen concentrate	8	100	13
Lime juice, from concentrate	1	4	4
Lemon juice	1	6	6
Orange juice, fresh	8	112	14
Orange juice, canned, unsweetened	8	120	15
Orange juice, frozen reconstituted	8	122	15
Orange juice, imitation (Awake, Bright and Early, etc.)	8	120	15
Tangerine juice	8	122	15

(continued)

Beverage Caloric Guide—*continued*

Fruit Juices—*continued*

Beverage	Serving Size (fl. oz.)	Calories per Serving	Calories per Ounce
Five Alive juice	8	114	14
Pineapple juice, canned, unsweetened	8	138	17
Acerola juice	8	56	7
Coconut water (liquid from coconuts)	8	53	7
Coconut milk (liquid from mixture of coconut meat and coconut water)	8	605	76
Blackberry juice, canned, unsweetened	8	91	11
Tangelo juice	8	101	13
Winter Hill apple-strawberry juice	6	88	15
Winter Hill apple-apricot juice	6	95	16
Winter Hill apple-raspberry juice	6	88	15
Mott's apple-grape juice	8	113	14
Pineapple-orange juice	8	126	16
Pear-apple cider	8	100	13
Pear-grape juice	8	110	14

Fruit Drinks

Beverage	Serving Size (fl. oz.)	Calories per Serving	Calories per Ounce
Orange-apricot juice drink, canned, 40% fruit juices	8	125	16
Del Monte pineapple-grapefruit juice drink	8	120	15
Del Monte pineapple-orange juice drink	8	120	15
Knudsen Hibiscus Cooler	8	94	12

Beverage	Serving Size (fl. oz.)	Calories per Serving	Calories per Ounce
Hawaiian Punch canned drinks, all flavors	8	120	15
Harvest of Nature fruit punch, sugar-free	8	8	1
Hawaiian Punch drink mix	8	104	13
Hi-C canned drinks, all flavors	8	120	15
Gatorade bottled drinks, all flavors	8	56	7
Hi-C drink mixes, all favors	8	104	13
Kool-Aid drink mixes, all flavors except lemonade	8	104	13
Kool-Aid drink mixes, sugar-free, all flavors	8	4	0.5
Tang drink mixes, all flavors	8	120	15
Gatorade drink mixes, all flavors	8	56	7
Country Time drink mixes, all flavors	8	88	11
Crystal Light drink mix, sugar-free, orange	8	4	0.5
Ocean Spray Cran-Tastic blended juice drink	6	110	18
Kool-Aid lemonade drink mix	8	104	13
Wyler's lemonade drink mix	8	88	11
Lemonade, from frozen concentrate	8	107	14
Crystal Light lemonade mix	8	4	0.5
Knudsen sparkling fruit juice, strawberry	8	75	9

Coffee and Tea

Beverage	Serving Size (fl. oz.)	Calories per Serving	Calories per Ounce
Tea, clear	8	2	0.3
Tea, instant, sweetened	8	86	11

(continued)

Beverage Caloric Guide—*continued*

Coffee and Tea—*continued*

Beverage	Serving Size (fl. oz.)	Calories per Serving	Calories per Ounce
Tea, instant, unsweetened	8	0	0
Celestial Seasonings Red Zinger herb tea	6	1	0.2
Magic Mountain instant herb tea	8	4	0.5
Postum cereal beverage	8	36	5
Coffee, black	8	2.7	0.3
Coffee, instant, black	8	1.3	0.2
General Foods "International Coffee," Irish Mocha Mint	8	67	8

Vegetable Drinks

Beverage	Serving Size (fl. oz.)	Calories per Serving	Calories per Ounce
Tomato juice	8	46	6
Tomato juice cocktail	8	51	6
V-8 vegetable juice cocktail	8	52	7
Carrot juice	8	93	12
Mott's Beefamato	8	97	12
Mott's Clamato	8	114	14
Knudsen Very Veggie	8	32	4

Beer

Beverage	Serving Size (fl. oz.)	Calories per Serving	Calories per Ounce
Augsberger	12	175	15
Beck's dark	12	156	13
Beck's light	12	132	11

Beverage	Serving Size (fl. oz.)	Calories per Serving	Calories per Ounce
Birell Premium Light nonalcohol malt beverage	12	75	6
Budweiser	12	150	13
Busch	12	156	13
Coors	12	142	12
Coors Light	12	102	9
Dos Equis amber	12	144	12
Foster's lager	12	120	10
Gablinger's	12	96	8
Guinness Extra Stout	12	192	16
Hamm's	12	136	11
Heineken	12	152	13
Heineken Special Dark	12	192	16
Hofbrau dark reserve	12	204	17
Hofbrau light reserve	12	144	12
Kirin	12	149	12
Kronenbourg	12	170	14
Lowenbrau	12	157	13
Michelob	12	163	14
Michelob Light	12	134	11
Miller High Life	12	150	13
Miller Lite	12	96	8
Natural Light	12	110	9
Newcastle Brown Ale	12	144	12
Pabst Blue Ribbon	12	150	13
Schlitz	12	148	12
Schlitz Light	12	96	8
St. Pauli Girl light	12	144	12
St. Pauli Girl dark	12	156	13
Stroh Boch	12	157	13
Stroh Bohemian	12	148	12
Stroh Light	12	115	10
Texas Select nonalcohol malt beverage	12	65	5
Wurzburger Hofbrau nonalcohol malt beverage	12	111	9

(continued)

Beverage Caloric Guide – *continued*

Wine

Beverage	Serving Size (fl. oz.)	Calories per Serving	Calories per Ounce
Champagne	3½	71	20
Dessert, sweet	3½	153	44
Port	3	134	45
Red table	3½	76	22
Sherry	3½	147	42
Harvey's Bristol Cream	3½	207	59
Vermouth, dry	3½	105	30
Vermouth, sweet	3½	184	53
White table	3½	80	23
Carl Jung dealcoholed white wine	3	20	7
Martinelli's sparkling cider	6	100	17
Masson light rose	3½	54	15
California brand wine cooler	3½	20	6
Taylor California Cellars Light	3½	55	16
Fu-Ki saki	1½	36	24

Hard Drinks

Beverage	Serving Size (fl. oz.)	Calories per Serving	Calories per Ounce
Bailey's Original Irish Cream	1	85	85
Brandy	1	69	69
Cordials, liqueur	1	97	97
Daiquiri	3½	122	35
Gin, rum, vodka, whiskey (80 proof)	1½	97	65
Gin, rum, vodka, whiskey (86 proof)	1½	105	70
Gin, rum, vodka, whiskey (90 proof)	1½	110	74

Beverage	Serving Size (fl. oz.)	Calories per Serving	Calories per Ounce
Gin, rum, vodka, whiskey (94 proof)	1½	116	77
Gin, rum, vodka, whiskey (100 proof)	1½	124	83
Jose Cortez tequila (80 proof)	1½	36	24
Kahlua	1	119	119
Manhattan	3¼	233	72
Martini	2½	152	61
Whiskey sour	3½	184	53

Soft Drinks

Beverage	Serving Size (fl. oz.)	Calories per Serving	Calories per Ounce
Quinine soda	12	113	9
Club soda	12	0	0
Dad's root beer	12	158	13
Shasta root beer	12	164	14
Hires root beer	12	150	13
Old Tyme ginger beer	12	160	13
Faygo old-fashioned root beer, sugar-free	8	0	0
Dr. Brown's orange soda	12	174	15
Shasta orange soda	12	128	11
Dr. Brown's cream soda	12	162	14
A-Treat cream soda	12	126	11
Old Tyme cream soda	12	160	13
Old Tyme apple soda	12	160	13
Moxie soda	12	180	15
Yoo Hoo chocolate drink	12	180	15
Bitter Lemon	6	96	16
Pepsi	12	158	13
Diet Pepsi	12	0	0
Coca-Cola	12	144	12

(continued)

Beverage Caloric Guide—*continued*
Soft Drinks—*continued*

Beverage	Serving Size (fl. oz.)	Calories per Serving	Calories per Ounce
Diet Coke	12	0	0
A-Treat cola, sugar-free	12	6	0.5
Dr. Pepper	12	144	12
7-Up	12	146	12
Diet 7-Up	12	4	0.3
Mountain Dew	12	178	15

Milk Drinks

Beverage	Serving Size (fl. oz.)	Calories per Serving	Calories per Ounce
Whole milk, 3.5% fat	8	159	20
Low-fat milk, 2% fat	8	120	15
Low-fat milk, 1% fat	8	102	13
Low-fat milk, 1% fat, lactose reduced	8	100	13
Skim milk	8	86	11
Buttermilk	8	99	12
Goat's milk	8	168	21
Eggnog (no alcohol)	4	171	43
Malted milk, chocolate	8	233	29
Chocolate milk, whole	8	208	26
Hot cocoa	8	218	27
Carnation hot cocoa mix, regular	6	110	18
Carnation hot cocoa mix, sugar-free	6	50	8
Swiss Miss chocolate milk mix, sugar-free	8	130	16
Nestle Quik chocolate milk mix	8	245	31
Nestle Quik chocolate milk mix, sugar-free	8	140	18

Beverage	Serving Size (fl. oz.)	Calories per Serving	Calories per Ounce
Burger King vanilla shake	16	340	21
Burger King chocolate shake	16	340	21
McDonald's vanilla shake	16	352	22
McDonald's chocolate shake	16	383	24
Hardee's milkshake	16	391	24
Dairy Queen chocolate shake, regular	16	710	44
Ovaltine, whole milk	8	221	28
Kefir, from whole milk	8	168	21

Miscellaneous

Beverage	Serving Size (fl. oz.)	Calories per Serving	Calories per Ounce
Ah Soy nondairy beverage, vanilla	6	142	24
Ah Soy nondairy beverage, chocolate	6	149	25
Soy Moo nondairy beverage, plain	6	98	16
Clam juice	8	20	3
Herb Ox instant beef broth	6	6	1
Herb Ox instant chicken broth	6	6	1
Mineral water	8	0	0
Pero instant cereal beverage	6	3.2	0.5
Tonic water	12	132	11
Coco Goya, piña colada mixer*	3	456	0.5

*1 piña colada = 3 mugs of Budweiser. Serving for serving, piña coladas are the most caloric alcoholic drinks in the world, tipping the scales at up to 450 calories or more each.

CHAPTER 7

The Psychology of Successful Weight Loss

If you have friends who diet all the time but never get slim, ask them how they imagine their lives might be when the years of salads and cravings and premeasured meals are finally over and they attain a stable, comfortable close-to-ideal weight.

Chances are they will tell you that on such a day their lives will become totally positive. They will be able to wear designer swim wear and tapered shirts. They will be their own best friends. In short, life will be as it should be.

But current wisdom on weight loss—as it applies to those who tend to over-eat—is that people are more successful at shedding weight and keeping it shed if they start thinking positively about themselves right now, while the pounds are still in place.

Easier said than done, of course. But many psychologists say (and psychology now plays a major role in the weight-loss world), that effective weight loss is easier when people banish negative thought patterns from their minds and replace them with positive ones. Kelly D. Brownell, Ph.D., of the Obesity Research Clinic at the University of Pennsylvania School of Medicine, has studied these negative thoughts. He divides them into four categories.

The first category he calls "Dichotomous Thinking." "Overweight people," Dr. Brownell says, "tend to split their lives into two separate compartments. They are either 'on' or 'off' their diets—never in between. We also call this 'light bulb thinking' because a light bulb is either on or off."

"For instance, I recently asked one of the women at the clinic how her diet was going," he told us. "She said it was terrible. It turned out that last week she stayed on her 1,200-calorie-a-day diet for six days out of seven. But all she could think about was that she had gone 'off' the diet once. She didn't think positively about the six days she was on it."

He calls the second category of negative thinking "The Impossible Dream." Dieters apparently set unrealistic goals for themselves and then feel guilty about not reaching them. "One woman told me that she was going to lose 50 pounds in time for her daughter's wedding," Dr. Brownell said. "The wedding was only a month away and she obviously couldn't have done it. She may actually have lost 20 pounds, but she would still feel as if she failed."

"The Awful Imperative" is the third category. Dieters, it seems, establish strict rules for themselves which, because of normal human nature, they will inevitably break. "They tell themselves, 'I will *never* eat chocolate cake again,' or 'I will *never* stop for fries and a milkshake on the way home,' or 'I will *never* buy a doughnut when the cart comes around at the office,'" Dr. Brownell says. "And when they fail, they can't forgive themselves."

Then there's category number four, "Dead End Thinking." It's based on envy. Overweight people fall into it when they focus on the unchangeable fact that some people seem to "eat like horses and still look like models." This form of thinking goes nowhere.

Why establish these categories? To provide dieters with mental first-aid, Dr. Brownell says. Whenever they feel anxious or guilty, they can stop and ask themselves whether their thoughts belong in one of the categories and, if so, can be dismissed as irrational.

Try to "Think Thin"

Sometimes, however, it takes positive imagery to reinforce positive thought patterns and make them more effective. Hypertensives lower their blood pressure with thoughts of Hawaii. Similarly, overweight people can, to some extent, get thin by thinking thin.

"We ask them to imagine themselves lighter," says psychologist Peter M. Miller, Ph.D., director of the Hilton Head Health Institute, Hilton Head, South Carolina. He believes that building confidence and self-esteem is more important, at first, than losing pounds.

"Instead of asking them to pretend that they are already at their ideal weight—that could be discouraging—we tell them to imagine that they are about 20 pounds lighter. Then we tell them to close their eyes and see themselves standing in front of a mirror with a bathing suit on, looking the way they'd like to look," Dr. Miller says.

"Then we ask them to imagine how it would feel to be shopping for flattering clothes, or to be working in an office or to be in certain family situations. It's important for them to visualize themselves behaving differently rather than just appearing different."

Images as mental tools are also important to Suki Rappaport, Ph.D., director of the Transformations Institute in Mill Valley, California. She believes that people with a positive attitude can make over their lives against great odds. To help her overweight clients she has created two images. For lack of formal names, call one the "nourishment pie" and the other, "the human tape deck."

If you're serious about controlling your weight, she says, draw a circle and prepare to divide it up as if it were a pie. Pretend that it represents all of the various ways in which you can give yourself physical or emotional nourishment. If you are someone who can't lose weight, that pie may, at the moment, be filled with nothing but food.

Dr. Rappaport asks her clients to identify every potential source of nourishment and tells them to give each one a proportionate slice of the pie. If they like swimming, they should give swimming a slice that reflects its importance to them. If they like films, theatergoing should get a slice. Using this image, Dr. Rappaport shows people, in a very positive way, that food isn't their only source of pleasure.

She also asks her clients to imagine that their bodies are cassette tape recorders and that each of their customary ways of responding to the world is represented by a different tape. She says that overweight people too often reach for the "binge" tape when they become anxious. Ideally, in her opinion, overweight people should get rid of their eating tape and come up with a tape that is more constructive.

"We try to say 'yes' to positive, life-affirming things, rather than 'no, no, no' to negative things," Dr. Rappaport says. "Then people realize, 'I could have gotten a great massage with the time and money I spent eating.' This approach gives people new options."

Clothes Make the Man and Woman

Clothing, interestingly, can have symbolic value for someone who is trying to lose weight. Max Rosenbaum, Ph.D., a New York psychologist, has found that men and women who have been losing and gaining for many years often accumulate a closet full of clothes of many different sizes. A man may have shirts with necks of 15, 16 and 17 inches, and a woman might have dresses from size 7 to 13 from "junior" to "misses."

"One woman we know spent her adolescence swinging back and forth, gaining weight and losing it," says Dr. Rosenbaum, who runs an obesity treatment program at the American Short-Term Therapy Center, in New York, which he and a colleague founded. "As a result, she never gained a clear image of herself. Her closet was full of clothes of different sizes, depending on her measurements at the moment, and these clothes prevented her from gaining a stable self-image. 'If I am fat today and skinny tomorrow,' she would think, 'then who am I? Which is the real me?'"

Dr. Miller's patients have run into the same sort of problem. He deals with it this way. "We tell people to throw away their bigger sizes," he says. "They've got to cut down to one size of clothes. We say, if they intend to keep their weight down, why keep those clothes? We know that as long as those clothes are in the closet, they will have doubts about their ability to change, and they'll be more likely to slip." In this way, clothes change from being a negative incentive into a positive incentive.

Yet another way to develop a positive self-image is simply to start reaching out to other people. "I tell my overweight women patients to start saying nice things to their husbands and children and start thinking positively about their friends," says Aileen B. Ludington, M.D., of Los Angeles, who once battled a weight problem of her own. "People find that if they can make other people happy, then their own self-image improves. I ask them to make a list of the things they like about their spouses and children. If you write things down, it's easier to visualize a problem. And it works for them. They come back with stories about how much their families are responding to them."

Fat Insulates the Psyche

Within the field of psychotherapy, there is an approach to solving weight problems significantly different from the ones mentioned so far. Many psychiatrists, for example, believe that overeating is self-destructive behavior and they treat it as a symptom of self-hate. Overeaters use food to comfort themselves when they are unhappy, the theory goes. They do so because it is less painful to raid the refrigerator than to unearth the emotional roots of their unhappiness.

"Food is a basic form of oral gratification, an immature method of finding security. And when people are agitated, eating helps them feel better," says Dr. Rosenbaum. "People use their weight as a defense against upsetting problems. Their fat acts as insulation against hurt."

"Staying fat can become very comfortable. The idea of losing weight and actually becoming thin would present a whole new set of problems," says Mildred Klingman, a New York psychotherapist and author of the book *The Secret Lives of Fat People* (Houghton-Mifflin).

"People who are overweight are very sensitive people," adds Dr. Rappaport. "They can sense dishonesty, and when they do, they retreat into a system that they have control over. They can control the size of their bodies. And their fat gives them a buffer zone."

Overweight young women often have mothers who habitually criticize their appearance, psychiatrists say. In many cases, the same mother once urged her daughter to "eat, eat, eat" for good health. This situation makes the girl angry with herself and with her mother. Overeating supplies an outlet for the anger.

"One young woman we know got even with her mother by overeating," says Milton Berger, M.D., who co-founded the American Short-Term Therapy Center with Dr. Rosenbaum. "She knew how upset her mother would get. There's a certain satisfaction to that, a vindictive satisfaction in triumphing over others. At the same time she is really only hurting herself."

Dr. Brownell takes issue with the emphasis of this approach. He believes that some professionals err in suggesting that the majority of overweight people have emotional problems and that they need to resolve their repressed conflicts before they can solve their eating problems.

"Some professionals tell people that they are maladjusted," he says. "So many overweight people fall prey to the idea that they hate themselves and that they are stuck in an immature stage of development. This is counterproductive."

Which technique, then, works best? The answer can only be that different therapies work for different people. But it's clear that change can't take place until each overweight person upgrades his or her self-image.

"Overweight people must learn to respect their bodies," Dr. Rosenbaum says. "That's very basic to successful weight loss. Overeating is closely related to poor self-concept. And when they begin to go through withdrawal, as all overweight people do, they have to say to themselves, 'I respect my body. I want to live.'"

CHAPTER 8

All about Fat-Removal Operations

Surgeon: First I'm going to put you to sleep. Then I'm going to make some tiny incisions here on your waist and each of your thighs and insert this suction tube and then switch on the suction and . . .

Patient: Will this hurt?

Surgeon: You won't feel a thing. I'll suck out all that ugly fat, just drain away your "saddlebags" and vacuum off those "love handles" forever. And when you wake up, you'll be down to a size 7 and won't have any scars or bruises or anything. You'll have to get rid of those size-13 dresses and buy some skintight jeans to show off the beautiful you. You'll want to wear a bikini on the beach and you'll get whistled at a lot and . . .

Such a fantasy surely danced in the heads of hundreds when the news first broke about suction lipectomy, the latest fat-removing technique imported from France. And, apparently, the dream of instant svelte dies hard.

Practitioners of the art (mostly plastic surgeons and dermatologists) have been trying to curb some of the wishful thinking, but the procedure's image as a "magic bullet" against flab and sag persists. More than 4,000 Americans have submitted to the treatment, and more candidates are queuing up from coast to coast.

The operation is the newest technique in an old trend toward "fat surgery," the radical tactic in the war on flab. It follows the intestinal bypass, gastric bypass, gastroplasty and a long list of variations on them all.

Their proponents are the first to point out that the procedures are for the select few—the seriously obese or, in the case of suction lipectomy, those with well-entrenched clumps of fat here and there. But the appeal of the surgical option is strong. Some people no doubt view fat surgery as a way around the brutal arithmetic of all weight gain: When calorie intake exceeds calorie expenditure, the result is fat, often just where you don't want it. For them, solving the caloric arithmetic is a long, hard road, and fat surgery is a waiting taxi.

Even with inflated expectations aside, the surgeon's answer to flab has always been overshadowed by looming questions. And perhaps the most compelling ones are those that come most readily to mind: Does the operation work, and is it safe?

Scooping Up Lipids

Darlene K., 33, of Andrews, North Carolina, wondered just that about suction lipectomy and then eventually decided to give it a try. "I'm four feet eleven inches tall and weighed only 100 pounds at the time of the operation," she says. "But I had saddlebag thighs and desperately wanted to get rid of them."

The surgeon anesthetized her from the waist down using local anesthesia (general anesthesia is often used, too), gave her intravenous Valium and completed the procedure in half an hour. Two hours later she was hobbling about, and in five days she was back at work.

She had to wear a girdlelike bandage for a week, and her thighs hurt for four days. For a month they were sore and bruised, and for two months there was numbness in one of them.

"I think it was worth the risk," she says. "My saddlebags are gone, and that's all that matters."

Donna C., 35, of Richmond, Virginia, got the saddlebag treatment, too, along with many of the same aftereffects. "The operation took two inches off each thigh," she says. "I wouldn't say that the results are cosmetically perfect, but I'm never going to have Betty Grable legs anyway. There's some slight waviness in the skin, which they say will eventually smooth out."

The Limits of "Magic"

So it seems that sucking away fat is trickier than it looks, as novice practitioners have found out. The surgeon first must make a half-inch incision in the skin at the least noticeable corner of the lipectomy site. Then he has to insert into the opening a foot-long metal tube (a cannula, they call it) about the thickness of a pencil, which is connected by plastic tubing to a suction pump. He moves the cannula up and back through the fatty deposits, between muscle below and skin above, slowly drawing out the fat.

"This seemingly simple procedure is not simple at all," says Joseph Agris, M.D., Houston plastic surgeon and co-author of *Suction Assisted Lipectomy Clinical Atlas* (Terrico). "The surgeon has to make sure that he maneuvers the instrument in the proper plane. He must have good eye-finger coordination to avoid severing blood vessels and nerves. And he has to remove just the right amount of fat from all areas to insure a symmetrical appearance. If he suctions away too much at any given spot, he risks creating a hollow that is impossible to fill and may cause an unsightly indentation in the skin."

It's this apparent simplicity that worries plastic surgeons most. They fear that it might entice a few money-minded but untrained colleagues to wield the cannula on patients who could get along with no fat removal at all.

That fear was recently voiced by none other than the American Society of Plastic and Reconstructive Surgeons (ASPRS). A Society report that cautiously endorsed the suction treatment stated, "This procedure could be over-utilized by quasi-practitioners or untrained physicians who apply it to minimal or inappropriate deformities for maximum reimbursement, thereby generating significant criticism."

Such a blunt warning doesn't come a moment too soon, for some plastic surgeons privately admit that there are some medical professionals now performing suction operations without the requisite skills.

Not the least of said skills is careful patient screening. According to the ASPRS, suction lipectomy is *not* for just anybody with a weight problem, and any worthy practitioner will make that clear to every candidate that comes along.

"The procedure is not for weight control and certainly not for obesity," says Samuel J. Stegman, M.D., associate clinical professor of dermatology at the University of California, San Francisco, School of Medicine. "It's for men and women close to their ideal weight, with good skin elasticity, who want to shed specific deposits of bulging fat (such as on the buttocks, thigh, chin and abdomen) which diet and exercise can't eliminate."

Most practitioners agree with these stipulations and would even tack on age limitations. Some use the suction procedure only on patients 45 and younger. Others set the maximum age at 35. After all, age is a reliable indicator of the suppleness of skin, a factor that could make the treated area look like normal human flesh or a fallen soufflé.

"The candidate must have excellent skin tone," says Dr. Agris. "When the fat is suctioned away, the skin has to shrink to the body's new contours."

And that's also a good reason for the caveat against using suction lipectomy to help somebody drop 20 pounds. The skin's ability to contract limits the amount of fat that can be taken from any one area at a time. It's theorized that if too much fat is suctioned off the back of the skin, it may lead to ripples.

Or worse. Too much fat removal and the patient could go into fluid-loss shock. For as the fat tissue is sucked out, the fluids trickle into the void and get drawn out, too. It's little wonder then that the better practitioners set limits on the amount of fat they'll remove in any single operation: three pounds or less per session.

Gauging the Gamble

But sometimes even with the right patient and the right surgeon things can go all wrong. This procedure has its risks like any other kind of surgery. Most people who have the operation are generally satisfied with the results and have few complications, but some wish they had let well enough alone.

"There are some complications that worry me more than others," says Kelman Cohen, M.D., chairman of plastic surgery at the Medical College of Virginia, in Richmond. "They're blood loss, fluid loss and hematoma [hemorrhage under the skin]. And, of course, the likelihood of these problems is greatest among unqualified practitioners." This is why Dr. Cohen feels this procedure is best done by plastic surgeons.

The ASPRS worries about complications, too. Their report on suction lipectomy mentions the possibility of skin dimpling (what they call a "cottage cheese" skin texture), fluid retention, pain, asymmetry in fat removal, waviness in the skin, pigmentation problems, scarring, skin sloughing (peeling away) and permanent numbness.

The worst possibility, however, is not on the list: perforation of the abdomen. Plastic surgeons say that it would be easy for an untrained and unhandy practitioner to push the cannula right through the abdominal wall.

Perhaps the most unsettling fact about the procedure is that it's so new that there's little precise data on the probability of complications. Plastic surgeons say the risks are within acceptable limits, but the unknowns nag nonetheless.

There are even questions about the permanence of the postoperative results. After fat is suctioned off, can it eventually come back? Can remaining fat cells enlarge and thus neutralize the surgeon's efforts? Will fat surrounding the suctioned area sooner or later crowd into the artificial gap? Plenty of practitioners would love to know. And since a suction lipectomy costs $300 to $4,000 (depending on the areas suctioned), many candidates would probably like to find out, too.

Bypassing Willpower

We know far more, however, about the forerunner of all fat surgery—the intestinal (jejunoileal) bypass. For over three decades surgeons have used it as a last-resort cure for people who are "morbidly obese," those weighing more than 100 pounds over their ideal weight. Thousands have undergone the operation, and thousands have been followed up months or even years later for post-operative evaluation.

The procedure's claim to fame is that it forces weight loss upon the patient by short-circuiting the anatomy. The surgeon accomplishes the feat by coupling the beginning of the small intestine to its end (a few inches before the colon), bypassing about 20 feet of its length. The excised portion becomes anatomical excess baggage. The result is that food can't be fully digested, and huge bundles of calories get expelled instead of absorbed. For most bypass patients, this means rapid loss of extra pounds.

It can also mean disaster. Several recent reports have condemned the operation because it creates more problems than it solves. They document a startling array of possible complications—liver disease, bone disease, kidney stones, protein malabsorption, infection, gallstones, inflammation of the intestines, nutrient deficiency, severe diarrhea, vomiting, even arthritis.

More to the point, in some cases the intestinal bypass has proved lethal. Up to 6 percent of patients die on the operating table, and the overall mortality rate may be much higher—mostly due to liver deterioration. Already at least 91 people have died from postoperative liver disease.

In the latest indictment of the intestinal bypass, a group of surgeons at University of Kentucky Medical Center, in Lexington, declare, "It is our contention that a 50 percent morbidity [complication] rate and roughly a 10 percent mortality following jejunoileal bypass are sufficient reason to abandon it as an appropriate operation for the morbidly obese" (*Surgery, Gynecology and Obstetrics,* October, 1983).

Getting around the Stomach

It's no wonder then that most obesity surgeons have switched to the less troublesome gastric procedures, what some people call stomach stapling. The operations—for desperately obese people only—are designed to ensure drastic weight loss by playing a surgical sleight-of-hand on the patient's stomach and appetite.

The trick involves partitioning the stomach with steel staples so that there's a small pouch near the top, the first stop for food on its way to digestion. In the surgical variation called gastric bypass, an opening is created in the side of the pouch and a section of small intestine is connected to it to carry food through the lower tract. The lower part of the stomach becomes a useless hollow. In a version called gastroplasty, a small passage is formed between the pouch and the much larger lower stomach. Food enters the pouch, trickles slowly through the passage and down to the lower stomach and bowel. Regardless of the gastric replumbing, the result is the same: The pouch prevents a large food intake and fools the patient into believing that a few bites are quite enough.

The deception works—most of the time. In a recent study of 167 people who had gastric surgery, Lloyd D. MacLean, M.D., a Quebec surgeon, and his colleagues report that 60 percent of the patients lost at least one-quarter of their preoperation weight. Twenty-six percent of them, however, were judged to have "unsatisfactory" weight loss.

Unfortunately, many of the 167 paid dearly for the lost pounds. "Malnutrition developed in a significant number of the patients," says Dr. MacLean. "The effect was mostly due to their reduced dietary intake."

Because of this complication, as well as inadequate weight loss and obstructed intestines, 71 of the operations had to be redone (*Annals of Surgery,* September, 1983).

Other reports detail a wide range of complications for gastric bypass—from infection to hair loss to blood clots in the lungs—and say that over 30 percent of patients experience them. They give gastroplasty better marks, but point to bone loss, stretching of the stomach pouch and bowel obstruction as the more serious after-surgery problems. And neither type of operation can claim a long-term mortality rate any lower than 1 percent.

"Gastric stapling hasn't stood the test of time," says William E. Straw, M.D., of the Palo Alto Medical Foundation, in Palo Alto, California. "I worry that the procedure, like the intestinal bypass, may eventually prove medically unsound. Such operations may be warranted for some severely obese people whose weight is life threatening. But in my work with the morbidly obese, I've found safer—but perhaps less glamorous—alternatives: They're called diet and exercise."

Body Sculpting without the Surgeon

Is is possible to shed specific lumps of body fat—to "body sculpt" —without surgery? Experts say yes—sort of.

"It's probably not feasible to spot-reduce deposits of fat," says Ronald Mackenzie, M.D., medical director of the National Athletic Health Institute, in Inglewood, California. "But it is possible to achieve an equivalent result. Through exercise you can strengthen muscles and improve posture so fat areas appear much less noticeable. And by a combination of diet and exercise you can reduce total body fat and thus enhance your overall appearance.

"All this is especially true of the abdominal area, where increasing muscle tone often means greatly enhancing a slimmed-down look."

CHAPTER 9

Dieters' Deficiencies

If you're a dieter—and surveys show two out of three people are—there's a very good chance you may be endangering your health, warns Peter Lindner, M.D., director of continuing medical education for the American Society of Bariatric Physicians (obesity specialists). You may be able to take nutrition for granted when you're eating like a horse, but it becomes critical when you start eating like a bird, says Dr. Lindner, who also heads the Lindner Clinic in suburban Los Angeles.

Researchers have found that immune-system response drops in people on very-low-calorie diets, says the physician. "In one hospital study, the researchers were interested in the changes in disease-fighting white blood cells when exposed to vaccine. What they found was that the immune response was reduced in those individuals on improperly administered ultra-low calorie diets, making them more subject to infection. That is probably one of the most dangerous aspects of very-low-calorie diets."

"A good balanced diet in the higher calorie range probably gives you all the vitamins and minerals you need. It gives you some leeway to play with," says Dr. Lindner. "Drop it down to 800 or 1,000 calories and everything counts."

In fact, according to the Food and Nutrition Board of the National Academy of Sciences—which sets our Recommended Dietary Allowances (RDA's)—it is difficult to get adequate nutrition on diets that provide less than 1,800 to 2,000 calories. Most popular reducing diets call for 1,200 or less.

Balancing a Diet

It's hard enough to juggle the four food groups into a nutritionally balanced diet when you've got a few thousand calories to work with. Dieters have a tougher task. They have to concoct three healthful meals with roughly half the calories they're used to consuming. And they start out with a handicap—they don't know beans about nutrition.

Following a diet guide may not help. Many popular diet plans are full of dubious nutritional advice. And most dieters know only enough to plan a 1,200-calorie menu down to the last morsel. Knowing calories isn't enough. You can create three low-calorie meals a day without ever straying from the candy counter.

Perhaps the most important thing to remember when you're counting calories is that it's the nutritional value of the calorie that counts. If you don't know the value of a calorie, you don't know what you're missing.

But Paul LaChance, Ph.D., does. Dr. LaChance, professor of nutrition and food science at Rutgers University, evaluated the nutritional content of 11 published weight-loss diets. He chose the 11 because they ran the gamut of popular weight-reducing plans—from high-protein/low carbohydrate to low-protein/high carbohydrate, with variations in between. They carried such familiar names as Scarsdale, Stillman, Atkins and the Beverly Hills Diet.

Using the RDA's as a frame of reference, Dr. LaChance and his associate, dietician Michele C. Fisher, Ph.D., R.D., found that most of the diets were low in thiamine, vitamin B_6, vitamin B_{12}, and calcium, iron, zinc and magnesium. Thiamine, vitamins B_6 and B_{12}, and magnesium were often at levels less than 70 percent of the RDA. One, the Beverly Hills Diet, supplied less than 70 percent of the RDA's for more than half of the vitamins and minerals they evaluated, and was so low in protein the researchers predicted it would lead to a serious protein deficiency over a long period of time.

And there's the rub. Most diets are protracted, if not forever. "Most people stay on a diet for a long time. After all, weight loss doesn't occur overnight," says Dr. LaChance. "If a diet lasts only two weeks, the vitamin and mineral loss is not going to be significant. But as far as I'm concerned, women are dieting all the time and may have other risk factors—smoking, contraceptive-pill use—that can affect nutrient metabolism. For them the loss can be very significant."

In fact, researchers studying otherwise healthy men found that even without those extra factors a prolonged low-calorie diet had a damaging effect on their health. One group, which had previously eaten over 3,000 calories daily, ate about half that for a period of six months. Even though they were eating more calories than prescribed by most reducing diets, the men suffered from depression, anemia, edema, slowing of heartbeat and loss of sex-drive. They also tired easily and lacked endurance.

Some weight-loss regimens, specifically those that are mainly protein, can lead to a potentially serious condition called acidosis, which also can occur on fasting diets. In one study, people fed a diet of solely protein and fat lost about two pounds a day—along with large amounts of nitrogen and salt in their urine. They suffered from the symptoms of acidosis, which can include weakness, malaise, headache and heart arrhythmias.

Acidosis can be remedied by adding as little as about three ounces of carbohydrate to the diet.

Needless to say, bizarre diets that rely heavily on one food—such as grapefruit—are going to be nutritionally bankrupt. Very-low-calorie liquid diets can be deadly.

Women are always going to have to pay extra attention to the nutrient content of their diets because of their increased needs for certain nutrients. "For women it's hard enough to get things like calcium and iron," says Cindy Rubin, clinical nutritionist with the Obesity Research Clinic at the University of Pennsylvania School of Medicine.

Women generally need more iron and calcium than men. "Many women are going to have to supplement their diets with calcium and iron," says noted weight and fitness expert Gabe Mirkin, M.D., who ordinarily doesn't advocate dietary supplements. "One out of four women between 12 and 50 is iron deficient."

Though an iron deficiency may eventually lead to anemia, it has its own immediate health consequences. "When you're iron deficient, even though you're not anemic," says Dr. Mirkin, "you can't clear lactic acid as rapidly as normal from your bloodstream, so you tire earlier at work and play."

"The problem with calcium is that it's scarce except in milk products—the first thing many dieters cut out. Unless you choose skim milk, dairy products can be high in fat and calories," says Dr. Lindner. "It's difficult to get adequate calcium without milk unless you want to eat sardines, small bones and all."

How food is prepared may also affect a dieter's nutrition. "If you're eating a salad that was tossed three days ago, vitamins are lost simply by exposure," says Dr. Lindner. "If food is cooked too much, you can lose more. Especially at risk are the water-soluble vitamins, such as C and the B vitamins."

One of those B vitamins is folate. Women are particularly at risk of developing anemia when they aren't taking in enough folate, which is found in leafy greens. A form of anemia occurs when there isn't enough folate in the body to produce red blood cells. Folate deficiency also has been pinpointed as a factor in an often precancerous condition called cervical dysplasia.

Studies have also shown that low-calorie and starvation diets can lead to an excessive loss of zinc, possibly as a result of tissue breakdown. Researchers at the Veterans Administration hospital in Hines, Illinois, found that weight-loss diets between 600 and 1,240 calories can be zinc deficient, depending on the type and source of dietary protein from which the zinc is derived. Diets that derive most of their protein from red meat tend to supply more zinc than those that rely on chicken, fish, milk products and eggs, which are, unfortunately, the main protein sources of many low-calorie diets.

If it all sounds discouraging, rest assured that the obesity experts understand—and have more than one solution to a dieter's nutritional dilemma.

• If you don't feel you can add red meat to your diet or if time and money constraints make it impossible to eat only freshly prepared food, you may want to consider taking supplements. "Theoretically, it's not necessary to supplement your diet," says Dr. Lindner, "but realistically most people don't have the knowledge or the time to do it right. Especially if you're a women, a standard multiple vitamin that contains iron, B_6, folacin (folate) and zinc along with a calcium supplement should help you make sure you're getting all of the 26 micronutrients you need."

• Learn the value of a calorie. You know there's a big nutritional difference between a 200-calorie candy bar and a 200-calorie protein salad. But even so-called diet foods aren't created equal. "Choose nutrient-dense foods," suggests Rubin. "For instance, eat broccoli as opposed to lettuce. Both are low in calories, but lettuce is mainly water. You're not getting the heavy doses of vitamin A you get in broccoli."

• Go for variety. Not only is it the spice of life, it improves your chances of getting all the vitamins and minerals you need.

• Plan your diet menu from the four basic food groups. "Each of the major categories represents certain vitamins and minerals," says

Dr. Mirkin. "Grains and cereals, for example, give you E and B vitamins. Fruits and vegetables supply C and A. If you take in at least 1,500 calories a day and distribute your calories over the four food groups, you'll probably be taking in the nutrients you need."

• Eat more calories. We've saved the blockbuster for last. By eating more, naturally, you're more likely to meet your nutritional needs. But will you lose weight? Yes, say the experts, as long as you burn up some of those calories through exercise.

In his book *Getting Thin* (Little, Brown and Company), Dr. Mirkin advises eating 1,500 calories a day—and using an hour of exercise to burn off 300.

There are some unique advantages to this plan. Aside from losing weight healthfully, you'll stimulate your metabolism to burn even more calories. "You see, diets don't work," says Dr. Mirkin. "When you go on a diet, your metabolism slows down. When you're lying in bed, not even moving, you burn 60 calories an hour. If you're on a diet, you burn only 50. If you exercise, you burn 70—without even moving. Exercise speeds up your metabolism 24 hours a day, not to mention suppressing your appetite."

Dr. Mirkin recommends picking two sports—aerobic dancing and biking, for instance—and working up slowly to an hour of each on alternating days. "I specify two sports because it takes you 48 hours to recover so you should rotate the stressors on your body," he says.

Older people especially need exercise as an integral part of any diet plan. "The two have to be together," says Dr. LaChance. "When you're young, your metabolism is higher and you can get away with more. When you get older, your body changes. Your metabolism slows, your lean body mass goes down and your propensity for adipose (fat) tissue goes up. You lower your need for calories so if you don't add exercise, you get fat."

CHAPTER 10

The Truth about Fasting

After he had suffered for six years with colitis, gone through more than 40 different drugs and an operation to remove gangrenous hemorrhoids, 34-year-old Jack Goldstein wasn't looking for any more trouble. But it came one day when his doctor said the time had come for surgery.

But the Michigan podiatrist decided on something to which his and most medical doctors would strongly object. He stopped eating.

Dr. Goldstein actually went on a supervised fast at a New York health retreat specializing in "the ultimate diet." The only thing that passed through his lips was springwater—no medicines, no vitamins, not even a little toothpaste paté on the side.

Six weeks later and 40 pounds lighter, Dr. Goldstein felt weak but "physically reborn," as he puts it. No, his colitis wasn't completely cured. But it was better than it had been in a long time, and without drugs. It would take years of careful eating and more periodic fasts to keep his problem under control. But Dr. Goldstein believes the fast gave his body the rest it needed to focus all its energy on healing.

That's something most of today's medical experts scoff at. They think fasting is useless, and that it can be deadly. Dr. Goldstein's own physician decided the improvement was psychological. And a biologist from Pennsylvania, who notes that fasting slows the growth of intestinal cells, says going without food should actually have interfered with healing and aggravated the disease.

Their conclusions, Dr. Goldstein says, "just show how little most doctors really know about fasting, and how little they care to learn." But even he admits the dangers of what was for him a last resort. "Just because it helped me doesn't mean everybody should or can do it safely. I don't think anyone should fast more than a day or two without proper supervision."

What is fasting? Is it safe? Are there any accepted medical reasons for doing it? The answers seem to depend on whom you ask. And there are many questions yet to be answered when it comes to any kind of scientific basis for fasting's reported benefits.

To fast means to abstain. "Fasting is a voluntary abstinence from any food or liquid that contains calories," says Allan Cott, M.D., a New York City orthomolecular psychiatrist who has used fasting to help schizophrenics. Dr. Cott is author of *Fasting: The Ultimate Diet* (Bantam Books).

While a true fast permits only water, some people drink fruit juices and vegetable broths. A protein-supplemented fast that allows 600 to 800 calories daily of a liquid-protein drink really isn't a fast at all, Dr. Cott contends.

A Tradition Rooted in History

Fasting has a long and honorable place in religious practice, political protest and, of course, alternative medicine. Jesus, Elijah and Moses all fasted 40 days and nights as a way to do penance and clear their minds. The only instruction they leave is that it be done humbly and privately.

British suffragettes and Irish and Indian nationalists all have fasted for political reasons. One of the Irish fasters lasted 76 days before dying. But, if liquids are given, a healthy, normal-weight adult can fast for 50 to 60 days before dying.

The longest reported fasts were by two patients treated at a hospital in Scotland, according to Nevin Scrimshaw, Ph.D., M.D., of the Massachusetts Institute of Technology. One was a 30-year-old woman who ate no food for 236 days and reduced from 281 to 184 pounds. The other, a 54-year-old woman, went 249 days and dropped from 282 to 208 pounds. Neither woman showed any significant side effects that could be attributed to lack of food, doctors noted.

There have been several deaths reported among fasting obese patients, Dr. Scrimshaw says, but in all but one case the deaths apparently were due to preexisting medical problems that had been aggravated by the weight problem, not fasting. The one exception was a 20-year-old English woman who in 30 weeks of total fasting went from 260 to 132 pounds.

On the seventh day after she had resumed eating, her heartbeat became irregular. Two days later she died. An autopsy revealed she had burned up half of the muscle tissue in her body, including part of her heart.

But a properly supervised fast would end long before such damage could occur. Such a fast could even have therapeutic value, slowing the gastrointestinal reflex and resting the body.

"You know that saying, 'Feed a cold, starve a fever?' Well, we believe that if you feed a cold, you will *have* to starve a fever," says James Lennon, assistant executive director of the American Natural Hygiene Society, Inc., of Tampa, Florida, an organization that advocates fasting as part of a total health program. "When you are ill, you're going to have a hard time digesting food, and that could make you even sicker. Animals actually have more sense when it comes to this. They know enough to stop eating until they feel better."

Skipping a few meals when you're feverish or nauseated is a lot different, though, from fasting for days or weeks to treat ailments like arthritis or colitis, says George Blackburn, M.D., Ph.D., a Harvard Medical School professor of surgery who has studied some of the physical effects of fasting.

"There are no known therapeutic reasons for a total fast, not even weight loss, because the dramatic change in body metabolism it creates could cause organ failure and disease, and the composition of the weight loss would be an unacceptable amount of body fluid and tissue protein from muscles and organs," Dr. Blackburn says.

Most of the benefits seen in fasting come from food reduction and weight loss, and could be produced much more safely with a prudent diet, he contends.

"It's true that eating, particularly overeating, creates major metabolic stress on the body. It can produce a harmful excess of adrenaline and insulin. Cutting down does lessen hormone stimulation and allows the body to feel better." Could it even help the body to live longer?

Researchers at the Gerontology Research Center in Baltimore found that rats fed every other day lived 63 weeks longer than their cage mates, who were allowed to eat all they wanted. They also remained more active later in life.

Dr. Blackburn agrees. "Fasting for one day isn't going to hurt you, and if these animal studies are an indication, it may be of some benefit. It's a longer fast that concerns me."

What Actually Happens When You Fast?

Fasting, like any diet where you eat fewer calories than you burn, forces your body to consume its own tissues to stay alive, says James Naughton, M.D., a professor of medicine at the University of California, San Francisco, School of Medicine, who has a special interest in fasting.

Normally after a meal, the body uses the glucose from the meal to provide energy to the brain and other organs. It also stores some glucose in the liver and muscles.

When you haven't eaten for 12 hours or so, the body begins to use the glucose stored in the liver. That supply, though, lasts less than a day.

The muscles then begin to break down their own protein for energy, and release amino acids, which are converted to glucose. This is the major source of energy for the brain and nervous system from the second to about the fourteenth day of a fast, and with it goes a large loss of salt, water and protein. (In fact, up to half the weight lost early in a fast is water that is quickly regained when eating resumes, Dr. Blackburn says.)

But as the fast and the breakdown of tissue continues, body chemistry changes. More and more fat goes to the liver, where it is broken down into compounds called ketones. After about three or four days of fasting, the body starts producing ketones for energy. The body slowly burns more and more ketones and less glucose, so that by about the twenty-first day of the fast, it's burning 90 percent fat and 10 percent protein. It continues at this ratio until it uses up its store of fat.

Then, the body makes a final fatal dip into its protein supplies in the muscles and organs. Weakened chest muscles and the inability to clear secretions from the lungs make pneumonia the leading cause of fasting deaths. Fatal heart arrhythmia may also occur.

There are risks at the beginning of a fast, too, Dr. Blackburn contends. "Protein and mineral losses are front-ended. They start after 24 hours and continue for several weeks. Short fasts of three days, a week, 20 days, tear the guts out of the body tissue and could lead to a heart attack or stroke."

Those risks exist for someone with heart disease, artery blockage or poor nutritional status, says Dr. Naughton. "But a healthy person seems to be able to tolerate protein and mineral losses during that time without much difficulty."

Both Dr. Blackburn and Dr. Naughton agree that kidney stones and gout can be a problem for some fasters, too.

But vitamin and mineral deficiencies are seldom a problem during fasting if someone is well nourished before he begins, Dr. Naughton says.

"Some of the water-soluble vitamins that are more short-lived, like thiamine, might become low after about four to six months, but most of us have enough reserves so that you don't see a vitamin deficiency state during a total fast. By the time one might appear, the person would be just about dead from his basic protein and calorie losses, anyway."

But some good things can also happen while you're fasting. Blood sugar and insulin levels drop, says Dr. Naughton. While they rise again when eating is resumed, insulin levels don't always go as high as they were before the fast, possibly because glucose-starved cells have become more sensitive to insulin. But you could get these same effects dieting off excess pounds, according to Dr. Naughton.

During a fast your blood pressure also drops, sometimes so much you feel faint. This is caused by an initial large water and sodium loss. But blood pressure quickly rises when the fast is ended, and any permanent lowering is the result of weight loss.

Hunger, the constant companion of many other diets, decreases by the third or fourth day of a fast. And the mental lethargy, apathy and irritability seen during periods of semistarvation are less prominent in total fasting, Dr. Naughton says. In fact, many fasters report a sense of well-being, euphoria and clearheadedness.

Some of these effects may be psychological, as voluntary fasters report them more often than forced fasters, Dr. Naughton points out. But others may be the result of altered brain chemistry.

Both Russian and British researchers have reported that fasting raised the level of serotonin, a neurotransmitter that plays a role in mood and the ability to perceive pleasure, Dr. Cott says.

And recently, scientists at the University of Athens discovered food deprivation blocks the brain's uptake of dopamine, another neurotransmitter. That finding was particularly interesting to Dr. Cott, because, he contends, the medications used to treat schizophrenia do the same thing.

"I've fasted about 300 chronically ill schizophrenics, people who would have ended up in the back wards of mental hospitals," says Dr. Cott. After about 25 to 32 days without food, 65 percent had improved enough to return to some degree of functioning and leave the hospital. Those who stayed on a vegetarian diet after the fast were least likely to relapse, he says.

Fasting to alleviate the pain of arthritis is a fairly popular treatment, especially in Sweden, where a one-to-two-week fast followed by several weeks on a vegetarian diet is offered at health spas. In two different studies, Swedish researchers duplicated this treatment in their hospitals. Both found that fasting did indeed significantly reduce swelling, pain and stiffness in many of their patients, but only temporarily. Blood samples taken during the fast showed lower levels of proteins usually associated with inflammation. " . . . fasting seems to have a fairly potent anti-inflammatory effect," researchers at the University of Uppsala wrote (*Acta Dermato-Venereologic,* vol. 63, no. 5, 1983).

Two people with skin problems did show some longer term improvement on the vegetarian diet, possibly because they were avoiding foods that aggravated their symptoms, researchers speculated.

Some people don't have a food intolerance, though; they have a food obsession. They can't keep their paws off it, and they fail miserably at attempts to diet. Fasting can help some of these people to lose weight, Dr. Cott says, because it truly does break the food connection.

"A short fast to quickly lose 10 or 15 pounds gives some of my patients the incentive they need to stick to a long-term low-calorie diet," he says. "They become very careful about what they put into their bodies. It becomes almost a rite of passage into a healthier lifestyle."

But it's no magic cure. Like any other diet, unless it's coupled with changed eating habits afterward, it's notorious for quick weight regain, plus a couple of extra pounds.

"Most people *don't* learn much about their eating habits when they fast," Dr. Naughton says. "People who lose 50 pounds slowly on a low-calorie diet, on the other hand, can learn a tremendous amount about what and how they must eat to stay thin permanently."

Fasting's not for everyone, even its advocates agree. And it shouldn't be for *anyone* without an understanding of its risks and competent medical supervision.

CHAPTER 11

New Help for Your Chubby Child

Baby fat is pinched, tickled, kootchy-kooed *and* grown out of, according to popular wisdom, which also considers it less harmful than diaper rash.

But researchers in the Bogalusa Heart Study found that baby fat is far from benign. In fact, they warn, it may be an early warning marker of atherosclerosis, a time-bomb disease that begins as early as childhood and is responsible for one out of every two deaths in the United States.

The researchers, who published their findings in the July, 1985 issue of the *Journal of the American Medical Association,* examined 1,598 children between 5 and 12 years old at five-year intervals. They discovered that childhood obesity was directly linked to increases in blood cholesterol, a fatty substance that clogs and damages the arteries.

Explains David Freedman, Ph.D., a member of the research team from the Louisiana State University Medical Center, "What we found was that the children gaining the most weight tended to have the largest increase in cholesterol levels, which led us to the conclusion that overweight is likely to be related to an increase in heart disease."

And statistically, it's the rare fat child who doesn't become a fat adult. Children often don't, as their mothers hope, "grow out of it."

Studies have shown that the longer a child is obese, the more likely he or she is to remain so. Only about 14 percent of all fat babies stay fat throughout their lives, but nearly three-quarters of all overweight teens become overweight adults.

Parents usually need little convincing that there's nothing pleasing about their child's plumpness—if they notice it at all. Unfortunately, parents are notoriously poor at judging whether Johnny is chubby. "They're with him every day," says James Sidbury, M.D., director of the program for obese children at the National Institute for Child Health and Human Development, in Bethesda, Maryland. "Usually the weight increases happen slowly. The thing that knocks them between the eyes is when the child goes from size XX to size XXX and they realize they can't put clothes on him anymore."

A pediatrician can provide a more objective judgment by comparing their child's height and weight against a growth chart, which ranks children in percentiles based on studies of height and weight distributions of large numbers of youngsters. A child who is in the fiftieth percentile for height, for example, is taller than half the children his age and shorter than the other half. If he ranks in the seventy-fifth percentile for both height and weight, he's probably big but not obese. But a child who is of average height and above-average weight is probably noticeably chubby.

Once you've determined your child is overweight, you're going to have to acquire some nutritional wisdom quickly. A child who is still growing can't go on the latest quirky diet and sweat it off at a spa.

"Adults can go on all sorts of crazy diets and their bodies adapt," says Kelly D. Brownell, Ph.D., co-director of the Obesity Research Clinic at the University of Pennsylvania, School of Medicine. "If you put a child on a radical diet, it can interfere with his growth. You have to be far more concerned about nutrition with a child."

Some children—only moderately obese or overweight babies, for instance—do not need to lose weight at all. For them, a maintenance diet is the best route. As they grow, height will take care of weight.

Parents should be aware from the outset that slimming down isn't easy for anyone, even children. But there are ways to make it less painful. Here's some of the latest advice from several of the country's leading obesity experts.

Catch It Early

How early? The experts agree: when baby begins to prematurely outgrow his swaddling clothes. Obesity is a problem that, like many killer diseases, has a high "cure" rate when caught and treated early: when children haven't acquired poor eating habits and parents still have some control over the food they eat.

It's also easier then. "A child under eight expects you to control him," says Warren Silberstein, M.D., a New York pediatrician and author of *Helping Your Child Grow Slim* (Simon & Schuster). "You control his bedtime, what he watches on TV, so there's no reason why food would be any different."

Parents tend to lose some influence over the eating habits of more independent school-age youngsters who, at the same time they have candy money also have little motivation to lose weight. "A nine-year-old doesn't care what she looks like," says Dr. Sidbury, who has worked with overweight youngsters for 15 years. "Frequently you're batting your head against the wall until they become interested in the opposite sex."

But while prom gowns and communal gym showers sound like strong motivation, overweight teenagers have a dimmer dieting prognosis than younger children. By adolescence, poor eating habits may be already a decade old and overeating may have become an emotional outlet, serving as solace for dateless Saturdays or poor grades.

Sandy Lieberman is convinced that it's never too soon. Her son, Timmy, weighed only slightly over eight pounds at birth. But by the time he was three months old he was tipping the scales at 19 pounds, about the same weight his older sister was at 15 months. "He had no cheeks and no neck," recalls Sandy, who also has three daughters. "When we brought him home, the doctor told us we could start him on formula when he could take three ounces. He didn't start with three ounces. He had eight. He didn't start with one or two tablespoons of cereal, he had the whole bowl."

The actual slimming down procedure for the hefty infant can be fairly easy, as Lieberman discovered. On the advice of her pediatrician, she simply diluted Timmy's formula to keep his weight stable until he grew into it at a year and a half.

Some experts recommend substituting low-fat for whole milk and emphasizing low-fat meals, vegetables and fruit for overweight toddlers. "Usually controlling dietary fat is enough," says Alfred E. Slonim, M.D., director of the Obesity Clinic, a program for children and adolescents at North Shore University Medical Center in Manhasset, New York. "Fat has more than twice as many calories per gram as carbohydrates and protein."

Your pediatrician should be able to help you work out a plan for your child.

Parents will probably have to start a program of behavior modification as well—for themselves. The Timmys of the world are rare ("A small number of these kids come out of the womb as hungry as bears," says Dr. Sidbury.) More common are the infants whose mothers associate every wail with hunger or use the bottle as a pacifier.

Remember: Food Is Only Nourishment

Studies have shown that infants whose parents respond to their crying with food later tend to associate all kinds of feelings, from sadness to boredom, with hunger. Food should never be a substitute for love or attention, nor a reward for a good report card or clean room.

"You want Johnny to do it your way, so you give him a cookie," says Dr. Sidbury. "It's easy. You hand it out. The better thing is to use affection as a reward."

Dr. Sidbury also recommends that mothers, when they can, breast-feed infants. It helps a mother become more attuned to her child's hunger pattern. "When you breast-feed, the baby stops when he's had enough. With an eight-ounce bottle, the temptation is to jiggle it until he's had it all. Some mothers never learn how much their child really wants to eat."

Go on a Diet Yourself

Research shows that it's likely an overweight child has at least one overweight parent. If it's you, be your child's dieting buddy.

In his program, Dr. Sidbury found that when parents diet along with their youngster, "the chances of a child being successful go up."

Sometimes it works the other way around. When Jeri-Jean Thomas decided to shed 25 pounds—at age ten—her mother, Carol, was so impressed that she took off 50. Her father, Andy, dropped 65. "I started after she had reached her goal," says Mrs. Thomas. "I thought, if she can do it, there's no reason why I can't. She was my inspiration." (See "A Success Story to Learn From" on page 71.)

Give Positive Support

If the unmerciful teasing of other children doesn't help, your nagging isn't going to coerce your child into losing weight.

"Twenty-four hours of that is enough to drive someone to drink much less eat," says Dee Matthews, co-author of *The You Can Do It!*

Kids Diet (Holt, Rinehart and Winston) and founder of Diet Encounter, a successful weight-control program for children in Palm Beach, Florida.

"If there's a food missing from the refrigerator, don't automatically accuse the fat child," says Matthews, who was an overweight child herself. "Don't tell the whole neighborhood your child's lost weight. I tell the kids, it's your business, it's your body. Tell the child you're concerned, that you want to help. But don't ask, 'Did you drink all your water, did you eat your salad?' Let them do 99¾ percent of it. After all they're going to reap all the rewards."

She encourages parents to allow the dieting child to take part in grocery shopping and meal preparation. It's often a break for the chief cook and bottle washer—whichever parent that may be—and a good lesson in responsibility for the child.

Keep Active

Most obesity studies have found that overweight people don't necessarily eat more than those of normal weight, but they are less active. Exercise has to go hand in hand with dieting.

But, like dieting, exercise programs for children have to be tailored to their special needs. "First of all, the words 'exercise program' connote something to people, usually pain and fatigue," says Dr. Brownell. "It's hard to get overweight people, even children, to exercise. It's not fun, it's boring and it hurts. But it's not so hard to walk to the store or take the dog out or ride your bike. Studies have found that overweight people who get involved in a variety of lifestyle activities—like walking and bike riding—have better results."

Use Diet Tricks

What works for adults also works for children. Eating slowly, eating only at the table and quitting the "clean the plate club" can help change bad habits.

"Give kids water between meals to fill them up," says Dr. Sidbury. "Don't feed them finger foods. It's easy to overeat. Serve only foods you have to eat with a knife and a fork."

Behavior modification is the underpinning of the obesity research program at the University of Pennsylvania. Dr. Brownell has written a comprehensive workbook guide on what he calls the LEARN program for weight control. LEARN is an acronym for Lifestyle, Exercise, Attitudes, Relationships and Nutrition.

Filled with familiar cartoon figures such as Garfield and Cathy, the 215-page booklet can help a dieter with everything from keeping a food diary to learning the basic four food groups. Among its suggestions:

• **Look for patterns in a food diary.** When do children snack? What are their favorite fattening foods? Do they overeat when they're feeling blue or bored or plopped in front of their favorite TV show? This can help identify eating triggers and high-risk situations that can be avoided.

• **Walk.** It's one exercise anyone can do. Many overweight children are embarrassed to exercise and may even find it too difficult. But a walking program can be adjusted for pace and ability.

• **Find distractions.** This is an easy one for children who tend to have good imaginations. When they're confronted by an "uncontrollable" craving for something to eat, encourage them to think about something else—buying a new, smaller-sized wardrobe, wearing a bathing suit on the beach. The craving usually passes.

• **Develop alternative activities.** It's tough to build a model airplane or ride a bike while eating a ham sandwich. Have children make a list of all the activities that are incompatible with eating so that they can consult the list when they get the snacking urge. Make sure they list only activities they would find enjoyable, because the alternatives have to be at least as satisfying as a candy bar would be.

For more information about Dr. Brownell's booklet, send a self-addressed stamped envelope to Dr. Kelly D. Brownell, Department of Psychiatry, University of Pennsylvania, 133 South 36th Street, Philadelphia, PA 19104.

Turn Off the Tube

Researchers at the New England Medical Center and Harvard School of Public Health, investigating the television-viewing habits of nearly 7,000 youngsters, discovered that the children who watched the most TV were more likely to be overweight, eat between-meal snacks and do poorly in school.

The scientists suggest that the prevalence of childhood obesity could be reduced and, in some cases, overweight could be prevented simply by reducing the amount of television children watch.

Fight the Food Myths

Number 1: Kids get fat on junk food.

Right? Wrong, says Dr. Silberstein. "Any child who is overweight is overeating all kinds of food. Parents make the mistake of thinking, if it's good for you it can't hurt. You have to cut down in balance. You have to understand that good food can cause you as big a weight problem as bad food."

Number 2: Kids won't eat foods that are good for them.

Wrong, says Dr. Sidbury. "No question, what a kid eats for a period of time he comes to prefer. This was seen when epileptics were still being given special diets. These were horrendous diets. Nauseating, actually. High in fat, with very little protein and carbohydrate. After two years, these kids no longer liked sweets. They wanted only high-fat foods."

If it's all they're served, the experts say, kids can grow to like salads and vegetables and shun anything sweeter than a fresh peach.

A Success Story to Learn From

Her name is Jeri-Jean Thomas. Most people call her J.J. She prefers it to "Fatso," which is what she was called when she was 25 pounds overweight.

Ten-year-old J.J. Thomas of Lake Worth, Florida, lost nearly a quarter of her four-foot eight-inch frame in nine months at Diet Encounter, a program for overweight youngsters started by a Florida woman, Dee Matthews.

Dee is no stranger to weight problems. At 16, she was built like a defensive lineman: five foot eight, 265 pounds. She gained and lost enough weight to create a half a dozen J.J.'s. Before starting Diet Encounter 12 years ago, at the urging of her family physician, she shed 100 pounds that she's kept off.

The program, which she developed with the help of doctors and nutritionists at Doctors Hospital in Lake Worth, was originally open to adults. However, Dee noticed one night there were more children in attendance. "It was heartbreaking," she recalls.

(continued)

A Success Story to Learn From—*continued*

"It brought it all back to me." And so Diet Encounter—for children —was born.

What makes Diet Encounter so special (and with an 84 percent success rate, effective), says Dee, "is that we give the whole responsibility to the child—with some help."

Children are urged to do some preplanning: setting a realistic weight goal and a target date, taking measurements and even photos. Dee has developed a well-balanced low-fat diet of about 1,500 calories that includes not only three meals but snacks. Most children attend her weight-reduction and exercise classes at the hospital.

They're encouraged to help not only with the grocery shopping but with the meal preparation. That was the toughest part for J.J. "It was hard to make my own lunch," she says. Parents are expected to cooperate by buying the food the child needs and by keeping temptation foods out of the house.

Dee's own battle with fat has helped her work out some dieting tricks for the thousands of youngster's who've gone through her program. Among them:

• **Sharpen your appearance.** "A lot of overweight youngsters don't care about their appearance, so along with being overweight they have greasy hair and clothes that don't match." A new hairstyle, better posture and clean, neat clothes can help overweight youngsters gain some of the self-esteem they lack. It's important, because the lack of self-esteem may even be triggering their overeating.

• **Buy clothes in the size you want to be.** "I tell the kids: Go to Fantasy Island [a nearby clothing store]. Buy an outfit you like in the size you want to be, put it on layaway, and try it on periodically. When it finally fits, take it home." Some children find it helps to keep the outfit hanging on a closet door to remind them of their goal.

• **Write letters to yourself.** The letters can help children get to know themselves better. Dee suggests that, at the beginning of the diet, children pour out their feelings about being overweight and then, as they lose, respond to those letters. "Answer questions like 'How do I feel about my body now?' 'What good things have happened to me this month?' "

• **Serve meals restaurant-style.** It's easy to reach for another helping of mashed potatoes and gravy when all the food is on the table. It's not easy when the portions on the plate are all there is.

• **Reward yourself with nonfood treats.** A bottle of nail polish or a new football are better rewards for an "A" in chemistry or for losing five pounds.

The hardest part of the program for most youngsters, says Dee, is, not surprisingly, the last five pounds. That's the battle J.J. Thomas is facing. But she's not worried. She knows she's going to get there. The rewards for coming this far have been too great to stop.

"The best part of losing weight for me is having friends," she says. "I used to be shy and fat and now I'm not. One kid in school told me: 'I didn't even know it was you.' I felt great!"

CHAPTER 12

How to Get Back in Shape

This chapter is for those of you over 40 who can't remember the last time you did anything more physically demanding than hike up your trousers or wrestle with your conscience—but who also feel anxious to do something about it.

For that purpose we've put together a primer on adult exercise, an informal A-B-C in seven steps that can help get you out of the starting blocks and back in the running. Included are tips on finding the right "soft" exercise, on staying motivated and on reacquainting yourself with long-neglected muscles. Our advice won't prepare you for a 10-kilometer race. But it might help you lead a more active, more enjoyable life.

Why should you think about a fitness program at this stage in your life? For two reasons. First, physiologists believe that exercise is the best natural age-reversing agent ever known. And second, they know that it's never too late to benefit from working out. Based on talks with a variety of exercise experts, here are some tips for getting started.

Step 1: Get a Complete Physical Examination

You may be eager to start your new exercise program right away, but it would be foolish to rush out, buy a pair of striped sneakers and begin walking or jogging at dawn. All of the fitness specialists we spoke with emphasized the importance of a physical for people who've been "out of action" for years. Even though one of the goals of fitness is to rely on doctors as little as possible, an adult's exercise program should start in the doctor's office. Says Philadelphia clinical nutritionist Steven H. Small, D.M.D., "We recommend that anyone who is over 40 or out of shape undergo a complete physical before starting any fitness program."

There are two specific tests you should ask your doctor for. The first is an electrocardiogram, which measures the regularity of your heartbeat and displays the information on a graph for the doctor to see. The second is a step test (or some other comparable aerobic stress test), during which you spend five minutes putting your feet up on a step stool one at a time. The doctor will take your pulse before and after the test; the lower your heart rate afterwards, the more exercise your body can handle.

Beyond that, a physical can help you tailor a fitness program to your needs. The doctor will probably want to know what activities you used to enjoy or would like to take up, and what your health goals are. If your doctor says you shouldn't exercise, one fitness coach says, ask why.

Step 2: Be Patient, Go Slow and Don't "Redline" Yourself

In other words, know your limits and don't exceed them. If you own a car with a tachometer you know all about rpm's, or the number of revolutions the engine makes per minute. You'll also know about the red danger zone at the high end of the dial, indicating that the engine is turning too fast and might come apart. It's the same way with your heart. It shouldn't exceed a certain beat-per-minute level.

The accepted formula for figuring out your own maximum heart rate is to substract your age from 220. If you are 55 years old, then, your redline zone begins at about 165. But that doesn't mean that you should push your heart that far. Dr. Small says that adult beginners should stay within 60 to 65 percent of their maximum heart rate. On the other hand, James A. Blumenthal, Ph.D., of the Duke University Preventive Approach to Cardiology program, or DUPAC, says that his older patients often reach 70 to 85 percent of their maximum rate safely.

"Safely" is the key word. "The first thing I tell people is to know your age," says Ben E. Benjamin, Ph.D., a sportsmedicine expert and author of *Listen to Your Pain* (Penguin Books). "Don't try right away to do things that you used to do. Start very slowly and go especially slowly when you try things that you haven't done for years. A lot of people try to come back too fast."

Step 3: Become Aware of Your Own Body

Many adults lose touch with their own bodies. They may look at their reflections every day, but they don't necessarily see the gradual decline of their posture or the slow shrinking of their range of motion. Grace Hill, an exercise instructor in Hanover, New Hampshire, has noticed that when she tells her older students to reach up as far as they can, many of them lift their arms only as high as their ears. It's not that they can't go higher. They just aren't aware of where their arms are.

"The first thing I do is to draw people's attention to their own bodies," says Hill. "A lot of people have become oblivious to their bodies. They've lost their kinesthetic sense—the sense of how their bodies move and feel. They have to be re-educated. We use mirrors so that people can see what they're doing."

Yoga and fitness therapist Gopal Bello, a staff member at a health clinic in St. Johnsbury, Vermont, feels the same way. He tells his students to stand in front of a mirror and candidly assess their posture. Does the head slump forward? Is one shoulder higher than the other? Are the feet parallel? There's no such thing as good fitness without good posture, Bello says.

People also tend to lose awareness of their breathing. "In the effort of trying to begin exercising," Hill says, "most people unconsciously hold their breath. A good teacher reminds her students about breathing. You can't have endurance without it."

Step 4: Choose "Soft" Exercises

When the experts recommend exercises for people past age 45 or 50, they rule out contact sports of any kind. They look for soft exercises that build up the body without punishing it.

"Water walking" is one of the most intriguing soft exercises we've heard of. It doesn't refer to any biblical miracle. It refers to walking, rather than swimming, in a pool. At DUPAC, older people exercise by *walking* laps in a four-foot-deep pool. Walking through water is a lot more strenuous than walking through air, but the buoyancy of the water all but eliminates the impact of the heel on the bottom of the pool.

Not that there's anything wrong with swimming. Swimming gently puts every muscle in the body to work, and it's recommended by virtually all fitness experts. Bicycle riding, either stationary or mobile, is another respected soft exercise.

Rebounding is another recently developed soft exercise. Bouncing on one of those mini-trampolines that are about four feet wide and stand about six or seven inches above the floor is something of a fad, but people say it's a novel, low-impact way to jog in place.

Along with the right exercises, a person should know which exercises to avoid. University of Wisconsin dance professor Judy Alter claims that many traditional exercises are not only ineffective but also harmful. She points out six "don'ts" of calisthenics: bouncing, joint locking, arching, swinging, fast exercising and overbending the joints. All of them, she says, can harm muscles or joints.

Whenever you bend over to touch your toes and then bob up and down—that's bouncing. It can cause some muscle fibers to tear. Joint locking occurs when you hold your arm or leg rigid by extending the joint too far. Arching just means arching your back or neck backwards, as in a gymnastic back bend.

Swinging refers to exercises like jumping jacks where the motion of the exercise depends on momentum and your muscles are mostly passive. The potential harm comes when you suddenly reverse the direction of your arms or legs. Fast exercise refers to rushing through a strengthening exercise and not giving yourself the chance to feel the exercise strengthen your muscles. Overbending the joints is what happens when you do a deep knee bend so deep that your buttocks touch your heels. It puts tremendous stress on ligaments in the knee.

One rule of thumb: If you feel pain, stop, especially when you're confronted by what Alter calls "ouch" pain. "When teachers or coaches say, 'If it hurts, it's good for you,' they are wrong," she says in her book *Surviving Exercise* (Houghton Mifflin). A sharp, stinging pain— the kind that makes you say "ouch!"—means that what you're doing is either unsafe or too strenuous or both.

Step 5: Learn to "Seduce" Yourself

One of the major obstacles to a new fitness program is inertia. It's the universal force that keeps you from getting out of bed in the morning and donning your sweat suit. Kelly Kessing, a staffer at Dr. Small's clinic in Philadelphia, recommends this strategy for outwitting inertia.

"You've got to seduce yourself into going out there," she says. "For instance, if the idea of walking intimidates you, just don't tell yourself that you're going for a walk. Don't pressure yourself. Put on your sweatshirt and your shoes. Tell yourself, 'Maybe I'll go for a walk, and maybe I won't.' Even if you still don't go for a walk, at least you'll have been up and moving for a few minutes."

If you're still intimidated, break the job down into smaller chunks and tackle one chunk at a time. "Walk ten minutes six days in a row instead of 60 minutes one day a week," Kessing says. "And if at first you don't succeed, forgive yourself and start over."

Step 6: Find the Right Program

When shopping for a fitness center, look for a place that has treadmills and other monitoring devices. And look for a coach who won't mind answering your questions about aches and pains, clothes and shoes, liniments and hot pads. "A compassionate coach can give a person peace of mind," Kessing says.

Step 7: Remind Yourself That It's Never Too Late to Benefit from Physical Exercise

Dr. Blumenthal's experiments at Duke University showed that older people can reverse a weak physique to some extent. His group of 24 people over age 65 exercised on stationary bicycles for 30 minutes three times a week for 12 weeks. By the program's end they had lowered their heart rates and recovered a degree of aerobic capacity they hadn't felt in years.

"There's some controversy as to whether older people can improve their cardiovascular health," says Dr. Blumenthal. "Our evidence is that they can to a certain degree."

Fitness therapist Bello agrees that older people should be more optimistic. "People very often feel that they just can't get better. They take it as a given that they won't be able to do the things they used to do. But we've found that people can recover a lot of the range of motion they used to have."

One woman in her 80's, he says, had stopped driving because she couldn't turn her head to look behind her. Exercise gave her greater neck mobility and she started driving again. Another woman regained enough strength to return to her daily housekeeping chores. A third woman rid herself, through exercise, of 30 years of lower back pain.

Exercise is also one of the best antidotes to the retirement blues. "One of the worst things that people can do to their bodies is to retire," Dr. Benjamin says. "When people retire at 65, they deteriorate very rapidly. They should work as long as they can. And if they don't work, they should fill up their lives in other ways, such as exercise."

Dr. Small adds, "We see a lot of people in their 60's who are realizing that their lifestyle habits haven't been very good. They want to talk about how to change. We even have people in their 80's coming in for fitness counseling. It's never too late. No matter what age they might be, a fitness and lifestyle program can make a difference in the quality of their lives from that point on."

CHAPTER 13

"Soft" Exercise—
Today's Safer and
Better Way to Get Fit

Excuses, excuses. When it comes to exercising, there's never a shortage. It's too hot. It's too cold. You're too tired. There's no time. You've got a bug. Your back aches. Maybe tomorrow. Maybe next week.

Maybe never, if you still think that exercise means gallons of sweat and lots of pain.

Fact is, exercise doesn't have to be hard work, says one fitness expert. "You can get in terrific shape with a fairly moderate level of intensity if you take the time to do it right."

And huffing and puffing aerobic exercise, such as jogging, isn't the only way to go about it. Instead, get into the action with "soft" exercises. In that way you don't have to pound yourself to a pulp or risk injury to gain the benefits. On the contrary, in some cases you won't even realize you're exercising at all. Not with activities such as swimming, dancing, gardening, Tai-Chi and others.

But your body will know the difference. You'll become flexible, more mobile, even more cheerful. Best of all, you'll reduce your chances of developing osteoporosis (a bone-weakening disorder) and heart disease.

That's what the researchers are saying and they have studies to back up the claims. In the Netherlands, scientists investigated the relationship (over a four-year period) between heart attacks and light physical exercise—mainly lesiure-time walking, cycling or gardening.

The volunteers were divided into groups who exercised for less than four hours per week, four to seven hours per week or greater than seven. Then they were further subdivided according to whether they exercised occasionally (less than four months per year), seasonally (four to eight months a year) or habitually (more than eight months a year).

The researchers found that those who walked, cycled or gardened more than eight months a year had significantly fewer heart attacks than those who exercised only occasionally or seasonally.

What's more, this reduction in heart attacks did not depend on the number of hours a week devoted to these leisure-time activities, nor was it enhanced by more vigorous additional exercise.

"This is of considerable practical importance," say the researchers, because "vigorous exertion may induce or exacerbate life-threatening arrhythmias [abnormal heart rhythms] in the middle aged. Those who find and take the opportunity to walk, cycle or work in the garden, all year round, are probably far better off" (*American Journal of Epidemiology,* December, 1979).

"The idea is to keep moving," adds Everett L. Smith, Ph.D., assistant clinical professor of preventive medicine at the University of Wisconsin in Madison. "Even a little bit is better than none, whether it's aerobic or not. Just 30 minutes a day of walking or dancing will help stabilize the rate of bone loss due to aging."

In fact, in one study, Dr. Smith showed that osteoporosis could actually be reversed with a program of moderate exercises. During a three-year period, those who exercised demonstrated a 2.29 percent increase in bone mineral mass, while those in the control group (who did not exercise) had a 3.28 percent decrease in theirs.

Yet, the exercises used in the study were so simple that they could be done sitting on a chair—movements such as sideward leg spreads, knee lifts, toe touches, arm lifts, sideward bends and others. Fact is, those are the same kinds of movements that you'd get in soft exercises such as dancing, walking, swimming or roller-skating, along with a lot more fun.

A Sunnier Outlook on Life

No wonder those who get involved in regular soft exercising have a sunnier outlook on life. Apparently, what's fun for the body is fun for the mind, too.

That was demonstrated in a study at the University of Wisconsin

Medical School in Madison. Doctors there supervised a program in which ten men (aged 61 to 84) with various medical problems walked 45 to 60 minutes twice a week for a period of 30 weeks.

At the end of the study all the men had increased their walking endurance by at least 90 percent. Their leg muscles were stronger and their blood pressure and resting heart rate had decreased, too—just what you'd expect from a moderate fitness program.

But there was something else that the doctors noticed. These men—who had previously been depressed and socially isolated—were now clearly more hopeful and less anxious. Complaints about their physical condition decreased too, and that could be because the men were either less depressed or because there was an improvement in actual physical well-being. Either way, the exercise program is what made the difference.

It also proves that you're never too old to start. "I have a patient who has just begun to exercise and he's 97," says Dr. Smith. "The important thing to remember is to gear your movements to your capabilities. And incorporate your exercises into your total lifestyle. Then there's less likelihood of dropping out."

That means collecting a whole potpourri of things you like to do that can keep you going whether it's summer or winter, workday or weekend.

In other words, you may want to garden or swim in the summer, but then be ready to pick up with dancing, yoga or roller-skating when the seasons or your interests change. It's completely up to you.

To help get you started we've compiled a list of eight soft exercises (some aerobic, some not). But don't let us limit you. Use your imagination. Soft exercises can be almost anything you want, as long as they're active enough to keep you moving but gentle enough not to pound you down.

1. Swimming is no doubt the ultimate soft exercise because you can condition every muscle in your body (including your heart) while cushioned by water, thus sparing the leg joints from continuous pounding.

"This makes swimming particularly good for people whose joints have stiffened with age or arthritis," says Zebulon Kendrick, Ph.D., director of the biokinetics lab at Temple University in Philadelphia. "When arthritis sufferers work out in a pool it actually helps to loosen up stiff joints. This increased flexibility carries over into the rest of their lives too, and perpetuates the progress made initially by swimming. What's more, swimming helps strengthen the muscles supporting the joints, so that they become less subject to injury."

Lenore R. Zohman, M.D., and Albert A. Kattus, M.D., agree. They also point out in their book *The Cardiologists' Guide to Fitness and Health Through Exercise* (Simon and Schuster), that swimming is one of the few exercises capable of strengthening the back and abdominal muscles.

Further, say the cardiologists, swimming can help counter varicose veins. "The improved muscle tone in the legs from swimming massages the leg veins as the legs move, thus helping to avoid venous distention [swollen veins] and varicosities."

Besides doing all those good things for your body, let's not forget that swimming is just plain fun. It makes you feel good whether you're gently paddling about or intensively swimming laps. Either way it's a worthwhile addition to your repertoire of physical activities.

2. Walking is probably the easiest of all to stick to month after month, because it's already a part of your life. The idea is to figure out ways of fitting more of it into your daily routine.

"Get off the bus two blocks early," Dr. Smith suggests. "Or park your car a half mile from work. Walk to the store when you only need one or two items. And most important, walk with your spouse or a friend. It's a wonderful way to socialize and share your thoughts."

It's also a super way to get fit. A brisk walk (about four miles an hour) is usually enough for cardiovascular benefits. But a slower pace offers its rewards, too. You'll improve your endurance and flexibility and also burn about 100 calories for each mile you walk.

3. Gardening is a seasonal pursuit for many people, but one worth including while you can. Rock gardens, flower beds and vegetable patches all need to be hoed, pruned and weeded, and that means lots of exercise for you. Bending, pulling, lifting and hauling can improve your flexibility and strengthen your leg, back and arm muscles. As if that's not enough, you even have something tangible to admire when you're done.

4. Yoga is one form of exercise that reaches every part of your body, inside and out, say the experts. It incorporates 87 principal postures and each one has a specific reason for being. But basic to all yoga is learning to breathe in a special, healthier way. "Proper and slow breathing, relaxation following stress, nothing hurried—these are the keys to each yoga exercise," says Savitri Ahuja, author of *Savitri's Way to Perfect Fitness through Hatha Yoga* (Simon and Schuster).

Yoga promotes flexibility and good posture, add Drs. Zohman and Kattus, and is also helpful in reducing high blood pressure and cardiac arrhythmias in certain cases.

83

And yoga can be done at any age. In fact, the experts agree that the older you are the more you have to gain from practicing yoga. To learn this ancient science you will need to sign up for a class (Y's usually offer them) or buy one of the many excellent self-instruction books.

5. Tai-Chi is a quiet ritual of slow gliding and twisting, pivoting and delicate gesturing. It is a series of 108 linked movements, each blending into the next, so that the entire activity is one long, unified pattern.

Tai-Chi is deceptive. It looks so slow and easy, and yet a lot is going on. Every part of the body is brought into play. With Tai-Chi energy can be controlled, strength balanced and vitality increased. And since it demands no physical strength to begin with, it's as good for the weak as for the strong, and for the young as well as the old.

To learn the ways of Tai-Chi you'll need to take classes, which are often offered at local Y's or in adult education programs. It's worth mastering.

6. Cycling gives you the most fun for your energy when it's done outside, around the neighborhood or through the parks. But it's just as effective if you do it indoors on a stationary bike.

This is one of those exercises that can be leisurely (like taking a stroll except that you're pedaling) or super intensive (till your thigh muscles scream for mercy). Either way, you gain the benefits, which range from firming up thighs, hips and buttocks to total cardiovascular fitness.

Whether you choose a rolling or a stationary cycle, it's important to get a proper fit. "The seat height should be adjusted correctly so that the leg muscles can function most efficiently and energy won't be wasted struggling against the bicycle," say Drs. Zohman and Kattus. "With your toe on the pedal, there should be a small bend at the knee when the pedal is in the fully down position and the seat is at the correct height."

Handlebars should be positioned so that the body is relaxed and leaning slightly forward.

To make cycling a part of your lifestyle, start slow and easy. Pedal to the store or to visit a friend. Better yet, get your friend to cycle with you.

On bad-weather days, set up your stationary bike in front of the TV or pedal in time to your favorite album.

7. Roller-Skating is not just for kids anymore. Gone are the skate keys and attach-to-the-shoe roller skates. Real enthusiasts wear leather boot-type roller-skates, which offer excellent support and comfort.

But before you invest in heavy-duty equipment, it's best to rent first. You can do that at any roller rink, and at the same time find out if this activity is truly for you. So far 39 million people have taken up the sport and have probably improved their health to boot.

According to the American Heart Association, roller-skating can promote heart health, muscular strength and endurance. What's more, roller-skating is a great family activity that can be started at an early age and carried on throughout adulthood. Best of all, it rates a 10 in the fun department.

8. **Dancing** can be just as much fun as roller-skating. Whether you dance alone or with a partner, or whether your forte is the rumba, the polka, the twist, ballet, jazzercise or folk dancing doesn't really matter. The idea is to flow, rock, sway, turn and sweep to your favorite music, all the while flexing, stretching and working your muscles, and your heart.

Fact is, some dancing is actually too much of a workout for some formerly sedentary folks, so choose a slow pace to begin with. It's also a good idea to sing along with the music. If you can do this, you know you aren't overdoing it.

So go ahead and enjoy. Whether you keep your pace slow and recreational or build up to a higher level of fitness, you can't lose anything—except perhaps, some stiffness, weakness, flabbiness and inertia.

CHAPTER 14

Stairways to Health

A few years ago, Sandie Folender of Creve Coeur, Missouri, decided it was time to do something about her health. The 39-year-old mother of two, a self-described "lazy person," realized that her cardiovascular system needed regular exercise, fast. So she started shopping for a training program that was right for her. On a tip from a friend, she found it: stair climbing.

"We live in a two-story house, and there are 26 steps from the basement to the second floor," Folender explains. "I started climbing them every day after breakfast, and I worked up to doing it for a half hour a day.

"For people who say, 'I'm not athletic,' this is a really simple thing to do. It increased my stamina and gave me lots of energy. I felt healthier."

Athletic or not, a growing number of people are discovering that plain old stair climbing can be a comfortable, effective form of exercise. Cardiologists, physiologists and even psychologists like stair climbing too, and they recommend it for people who want to lose weight, strengthen their heart, control diabetes or just firm up their leg muscles and derriere. And stair climbing is a potent way to peel off a few pounds without really setting aside time for exercise. If you walked up and down a mere two flights of stairs a day, instead of taking elevators or escalators, you would lose an additional six pounds or more over the course of a year, according to Kelly D. Brownell, Ph.D., a University of Pennsylvania psychologist who helps people lose weight.

The number of calories that you spend climbing stairs varies depending on how much you weigh, how fast you climb or if you're carrying a load. But Lenore R. Zohman, M.D., director of cardiac rehabilitation of Montefiore Hospital and Medical Center in New York City, estimates that a 110-pound woman climbing stairs at a comfortable pace would spend about five calories a minute, and a 175-pound man would spend about eight calories a minute. Those figures would roughly double if you take two steps at a time.

Compared to other forms of exercise, stair climbing, minute for minute, stacks up pretty well. "Using stairs produces a surprisingly large expenditure of energy," says Dr. Brownell. "Even larger than that for such strenuous activities as jogging, swimming, cycling and calisthenics" (*American Journal of Psychiatry,* December, 1980).

A study conducted in Finland a few years ago demonstrated that regular stair climbing can help you lose weight. Tests conducted by an insurance company there showed that men who climbed about 25 flights of stairs during the course of a day lost a "significant" amount of weight after only 12 weeks. And climbing those stairs took surprisingly little time. The average, comfortable climbing rate of those men—who were between the ages of 17 and 64—was 100 steps a minute. At that speed, climbing a flight of stairs (at 10 steps to a flight) would take only six seconds.

Not surprisingly, stair climbing seems to be good for the heart. In England, a study of almost 17,000 male civil-service workers between the ages of 40 and 64 showed the frequent stair climbing was one of the vigorous activities that seemed to protect against heart attack (*Lancet,* February 17, 1973).

Another study of the men who work on England's double-decker buses also illustrated the value of stair climbing, according to Dr. Brownell. The conductors on the buses, whose job required them to climb the staircases at the back of the bus many times while escorting passengers to the upper level, were less likely to suffer heart attacks than the drivers, who sat down all day.

People who climb five or more flights of stairs a day apparently have a better chance of avoiding a heart attack than people who climb less than that. A couple of years ago a professor of epidemiology at Stanford University, Ralph S. Paffenbarger, M.D., selected five flights as a cutoff point for predicting who will suffer a heart attack and who won't.

Dr. Paffenbarger wanted to find out if men who are physically active really do have less chance of a heart attack. So he sent questionnaires to 16,936 Harvard University alumni who had entered the college between 1916 and 1950. He inquired about the condition of their heart and asked how many flights of stairs they climbed per day, how many city blocks they walked, and how often they engaged in either light or strenuous sports. He found that the men who climbed fewer than five flights of stairs a day had a 25 percent greater chance of a heart attack than those who climbed more than five flights a day. (*American Journal of Epidemiology,* vol. 108, 1978).

The study doesn't mean that simply climbing 50 steps a day will help you avoid a heart attack, explained Dr. Paffenbarger. People who climb that many stairs are usually physically active in many other ways, and therefore have healthier hearts. But that's still saying a lot, and Dr. Paffenbarger highly recommends stair climbing as part of a more active lifestyle. "I always climb stairs," he says. "I never use the elevator. I used to work on the seventh floor and climbed six flights of stairs two or three times a day."

Stair climbing is just as good for your leg muscles as it is for your heart, if not better. Every time you lift your legs, you're fighting both gravity and inertia, and the winners of that battle are the muscles in your legs and buttocks.

"Stair climbing is a natural choice for supplementing a fitness program either to maintain your current level of fitness or to increase it. The real benefit is strengthening your leg muscles," says Gary Yanker, a New York lawyer and walking enthusiast who has written *The Complete Book of Exercise Walking* (Contemporary Books), in which he devotes a chapter to the art and science of climbing stairs. "The leg muscles respond terrifically to walking up any kind of incline," Yanker says.

Climbing stairs can also be good medicine for people suffering from diabetes. In Augusta, Maine, where the snow piles up very deep in the winter and lots of older people find themselves housebound, Mark La Pointe, a public health advisor with the Maine Diabetes Control Project, needed a way for diabetics to find exercise in the winter — exercise that is crucial to diabetes management. So La Pointe turned to stair climbing.

"If they have an exercise bicycle, that's fine," says La Pointe. "But for people who don't we recommended just walking up and down the stairs. That'll stimulate insulin production and get their heartbeat up and maybe help them lose some weight. Stairs are very handy. Almost everyone has them, and they're really good for the elderly who can't put on a sweatsuit and engage in intense exercise."

Stairs are handy, indeed. They're probably the most overlooked physical fitness resource in America. Every staircase at home or in public is a potential "indoor fitness center." With today's mammoth two-tier malls, there are plenty of opportunities to climb.

But, statistically, hardly anyone chooses the stairs. Only about 7 percent of all men and 5 percent of all women pick the stairs over the elevator when both are available, and overweight people use them only about 1 or 2 percent of the time. Most people wait for the elevator to arrive even when it's obvious that the stairs would be faster.

Those were the figures that Dr. Brownell came up with. As a psychologist, he specializes in motivating overweight people to shed pounds by exercising. Experience has taught him that very few people stick to a formal exercise program, so he went looking for ways that people could work in a little exercise without changing their routines very much. He wondered if stair climbing would do the job.

Peeking at Pedestrians

To find out whether his patients would tend to resist or comply with suggestions about climbing stairs, Dr. Brownell first studied the ways that people ordinarily use stairs. He and other professors and a few students took up observation posts at a train station (where there were 18 steps), a bus station (24 steps) and a multilevel shopping mall (30 steps) in downtown Philadelphia. They made notes about who used the stairs and how often they used them. Over a period of months they ran two tests and watched 45,694 people. In the first test, only 6.3 percent of the people took the stairs, and in the second test, only 11.6 percent did.

The figures were discouraging but Dr. Brownell and his team did not give up. They commissioned Tony Auth, a political cartoonist for the *Philadelphia Inquirer,* to draw a sign that could be posted next to the stairways and would encourage people to use them. Auth made two drawings side by side, one of a feeble heart riding up an escalator and another of a muscular heart running up the stairs. Next to the drawings he wrote the caption: "Your Heart Needs Exercise, Here's Your Chance."

After the sign went up, the proportion of people using the stairs shot up to 14.4 percent in the first test and 18.3 percent in the second. Dr. Brownell decided that a fair number of his patients and people like them would take the stairs if reminded.

"We were looking for a way for people to include a little exercise in their routine activities and we found that using stairs instead of elevators was a terrific way of doing that. We're not pushing it as a form of training, but it's an easy way to exercise more. There are so many opportunities to climb stairs," says Dr. Brownell.

There are also very few excuses for not climbing stairs. "With walking, you usually have to spend an hour doing it, and when it's too cold or wet, you don't want to do it. My friends who walk usually quit in the winter and go back to it in spring. But there's no excuse for not climbing stairs and it's an easier habit to get into," says Folender.

If you enjoy stair climbing and want to turn it into a tougher workout, you'll find that it can be as rigorous as you make it.

One approach, which will get your heart and lungs going hard enough to benefit the cardiovascular system, would be a 20- to 30-minute workout combining stair climbing with interludes of level walking. For optimum benefit, this should be done at least three times a week.

Gary Yanker, in his book, describes stair climbing routines that take between 15 minutes and an hour. Roy Shephard, M.D., Ph.D., director of the school of physical and health education at the University of Toronto, says that an effective fitness program for a busy executive might be to run up three flights of stairs, taking two steps at a time, and repeat that nine or ten times a day.

If you get tired of climbing the same old steps, you can always find a way to vary the routine. Fitness expert and author Bonnie Prudden offers a few tips on making stair climbing more fun, in her book *How to Keep Your Family Fit and Healthy* (Reader's Digest Press). She suggests stair climbing to music, and she says you can get a good workout on the stairs in only about three minutes.

One word of caution: Even normal stair climbing can be surprisingly taxing and fitness experts advise working up to it slowly. If you work on the fifth floor of an office building, for instance, you might start by taking the elevator to the fourth floor, and walk up the last flight. Do that for a week, then walk up from the third floor, and so on. Of course, if you have a large number of steps to ascend, you may wish to walk around on one level for a while between flights.

One more word of caution: If you start stair climbing, you may never be willing to deal with slow, crowded lifting machines again. "It has made me too impatient to wait for an elevator," says Folender, "and even when I take an escalator, I run up it."

Rodale Press, Inc., publishes PREVENTION®, the better health magazine.
For information on how to order your subscription,
write to PREVENTION®, Emmaus, PA 18049.